Binge!

Dr. Ronald Jay Cohen

Binge!

It's not a state of hunger . . .

It's a state of mind.

Macmillan Publishing Co., Inc.
New York

Collier Macmillan Publishers
London

Macmillan Publishing Co., Inc.
866 Third Avenue, New York, N.Y. 10022
Collier Macmillan Canada, Ltd.

Library of Congress Cataloging in Publication Data
Cohen, Ronald Jay.
    Binge.
      1. Obesity—Psychological aspects.   I. Title.
RC552.025C63   616.3'98'0019   78-27364
ISBN 0-02-526950-X

First Printing 1979

Designed by Jack Meserole

Printed in the United States of America

This book is gratefully dedicated to my patients,
whose awareness, actions, and positive attitude changes
inspired me to write it.

Contents

you will · Midtown distressway · Beautiful binger · Churn! Churn! Churn! · Things are too good · Through another's eyes · I know my rights! · Just a taste · Deprivation · Hibernation · Procrastination · Bad taste · Love thy parents · Great expectations · Eating for two · Nibbling · London bridge · Penitence · Free for all · Black magic · Spellbound · Dentist chair · Red light, green light · Cannibals · Hearts and flowers · Crumbs · Office in the kitchen · Binge bingo · Rationalization · Charades · Miracle on Thirty-third Street

4

Breaking the binge: Awareness training

Eating awareness quizzes I and II · Calorie accountant · Feelings accountant · Demolition derby · Stop, look, and listen · Truth and consequences · What's wrong with this picture? · Is the price right? · Test of strengths · Gourmet · *Person*al touch · Fencing · Kentucky doily · Gag · Bridge · New math · 7 minutes in heaven · Kiss my 200s goodbye · Contagious outlooks · Stitch-in-time · Excess baggage · Bayonne, New Jersey · Reward or consolation? · What's important to me? · I am loved . . .

5

Breaking the binge: Action strategies

Calorie countdown · Student-exchange program · Let's make some deals · Once can be enough · Discrimination · Anticipation · Competing activities · *Person*al growth · 18½-minute gap · Glutton for punishment · Slowly but surely · Figure skating · Take out the garbage! · Anti-automation · Grab bag · Tag · Say "cheese" I · Say "cheese" II · Taking a dip · Hospitality personality · Speak your piece · LSD trip · Home-base ball · Chicken! · Go fish! · Hot potato! · Spin the bottle · Orange bowl · Happy D-A-E-S · Follow the leader · Tight places, smiling faces · Bathing beauty but no contest · Person to person · Simon says · Because I'm worth it · Blind man's brush · Out of

Acknowledgments

Over the years my parents, Edith and Harold Cohen, have freely shared much of their knowledge and insights on the subjects of dieting, binging, and eating awareness techniques and—in the context of this book—I am profoundly grateful. My grandfather, the late Mr. Hyman Schneider, had a wonderfully contagious sense of humor and I must also thank him for his contribution to my development, growth, and success as a clinical psychologist.

RONALD JAY COHEN

November 11, 1978
New York, N.Y.

Binge:

I

Some plain talk

about it

What is a binge?

A binge is not a state of hunger . . . it's a state of mind. It is a feeling of being out of control, a feeling of helplessness in which all normal priorities are somehow abandoned. A binge is loneliness, depression, frustration, anger, rage, alienation, and self-pity. It is a searching for something that you want very much but doubt you will get. It is a craving. It is an emptiness. A binge is a half gallon of ice cream, a pound of cake, a package or two or three of cookies, a bag or two of potato chips, or any combination thereof. It is an undisciplined self-indulgence engaged in by the young and the old, the rich and the poor, the fat and the slim. A binge is one of the few things in life you start out doing fully aware you will feel worse when you are done. A binge perpetuates itself: The bad feelings it produces lays the foundation for the next binge. A binge is something that no person or power on earth can stop once it begins—except you.

Why do people binge?

As infants we learned that a feeling of tension in our stomach (hunger) could be relieved by eating. As we grew up, this simple relationship between tension reduction and food consumption was reinforced thousands of times. Moreover, we learned to enjoy eating not only as a tension-reduction activity, but also as one that was pleasing in its own right. We were even rewarded with sweets and other foods by our parents. For many of us, food was paired with love. The tension-reduction value of food, the inherently pleasing nature of eating, and the inevitable pairing of food with love and nurturance should make one simple fact abundantly clear: Hunger is only one of many reasons why people eat.

As we enter adulthood we begin to experience emotions that can, like hunger, generate tension states in the stomach as well as other places throughout the body. Jealousy, anger, frustration, fatigue, boredom, and loneliness are just some of the feeling states that can generate such tension. Perhaps the person whose weight remains relatively stable is one who can correctly discriminate and respond effectively to tension-producing states. If such a person felt fatigued, he or she might lie down and rest; if bored, he or she might turn on the television, pick up a book, crochet, etc. Unfortunately, many of us are not very good "discriminators" of our feelings. We are not in touch with ourselves enough to discriminate, for example, anger from frustration. The danger in not being a good discriminator is that almost all bad feelings become associated with that most primitive bodily state of tension—hunger. In times of stress the "psychological shorthand" that causes us to experience a false sense of hunger interacts with other needs, such as our need to quell the stress and our need for love and nurturance. The result of all of these forces is that eating becomes our "old faithful" response to combat stress or console ourselves. And if one dollar is good, ten dollars is ten times as good, right?

The specific factors that trigger a binge will differ from person to person and from situation to situation. There are twenty-one common types of binges (discussed later). But the one common factor that runs through each is some sort of emotional tension.

How can a binge be stopped?

Ask someone who has ever binged, "What do you binge on?" and the answer will probably be, "Anything" or "Everything I can lay my hands on." This is probably not true. Most people have a very narrow range of foods on which they will binge. How many people do you know, for example, who binge on salmon croquettes? Knowing that there are relatively few foods used for binges, weight experts and weight-control organizations typically advise their clientele to keep problem foods such as ice cream, cake, and candy out of the house altogether. As a graduate student in clinical psychology learning behavioral techniques for controlling weight, I too was taught that problem foods should be kept out of the house—or at least hidden from view. However, clinical experience has proven to me that this is a very naïve solution to a very complex problem. Husbands, wives, children, grandparents, and other members of a household all have varied food preferences and needs. It becomes unrealistic and unfair to boycott one food grouping in such a household. But even if an individual is living alone there is still one very basic problem with the "keep it out of the house" solution: You are going to be exposed to chocolate, candy, cake, ice cream, etc. every day of your life whether you are at work, in the street, at a neighbor's house, vacationing, attending Aunt Bertha's wedding, and so on. You must, therefore, learn to cut down your intake of these problem foods, *not* cut them out.

Some people, particularly those who fashion themselves to be "foodaholics," seem to be able to maintain a weight loss through a program of total abstinence from certain classes of food. However, these people do not lead enviable lives. Clinical interviewing reveals that they frequently walk around feeling very deprived and somehow "different" than "normal" people. Besides feeling different, people who go the total abstinence route seldom stay totally abstinent from anything. The consequences of total abstinence come in the form of severe anxiety attacks when they put a teaspoon of mayonnaise on a sandwich or overwhelming guilt when they occasionally buy (or even take a taste of) an ice cream cone. The foodaholic's approach to the problem of the binge is a foolaholic's approach; it dooms the individual to a life of guilt, envy, and deprivation. The only realistic way to cope with and win the battle of the binge is to cut down—not out.*

How does one cut down? From our definition of a binge and our discussion as to why people binge, you should suspect that stopping is a matter of stopping the negative feelings associated with the binge and stripping food of its association with love and nurturance. However, there is more to binge-breaking than that. There are three crucial elements to winning the battle: awareness, action, and attitude. This book describes the "AAA" method of binge-breaking which consists of Awareness training, Action strategies, and Attitude change.

AWARENESS Contrary to what you might think, a binge is not a reflex action like a knee-jerk. It is a consciously chosen act that has both conscious and unconscious elements. Sometimes a binge occurs after a person has been on a diet for a while and they are just beginning to look good and get compliments. There is something very threatening about losing weight (frequently the threat involves a fear of sex or a fear of promiscuity), and the binge serves as a convenient mechanism to return to the safe status quo. Because a binge is not a reflex, it can be broken by a keen awareness of food intake as well as of the conscious and unconscious factors operating within. The first step of the AAA binge-breaking program is Awareness training. This training begins in Chapter 4. It is designed to help you identify the types of binges you indulge in and the binge games you play.

ACTION Unfortunately, too many Americans honestly believe they are taking constructive action against their problem eating habits by merely going on some kind of a diet. And every few years, like clockwork, there is some miracle drink, powder, or diet plan offered as the panacea to weight loss. These so-called miracle solutions have ranged from tap water to liquid

---

* We will have more to say about the myth of "foodaholism" in Chapter 6.

protein, from grapefruit to injections of pregnant women's urine and beyond. Predictably, thousands of people have lost weight on each of these diet regimens only to put the weight back on in time for the next fad diet. The latest diet craze in the New York area is one which, simply stated, claims that certain foods "burn off" certain other foods. Diet-conscious New Yorkers may lose some weight on that diet (just as they lost weight on the protein diet the year before, the water diet the year before that, etc.), but it probably won't be because tuna fish has the power to "burn off" breadcrumbs; it will be because they have reduced their caloric intake. What will the next fad diet be and how long will it take for its novelty to wear off? How many times must the public be duped before it accepts the fact that no scientifically acceptable evidence has ever proven that *permanent* weight loss can be achieved through any of the fad diets? When will persons with problem eating habits accept the fact that in order to truly gain control of their eating, they must first gain control of their lives?

Because a binge is a state of mind and not a state of hunger, what is needed to break binging habits are positive Action skills, *not simply a diet*. The serious binge-breaker is the one who realizes that people waiting for the miracle weight-loss method will probably wait with their weight into old age (or more probably die young as a result of cardiovascular disorders, diabetes, or any of the numerous other serious diseases that have been found to be more common in overweight persons). The serious binge-breaker is the one who accepts the fact that there are no miracle weight-loss drugs, diets, or methods and there probably never will be. Fortunately, in the serious business of binge-breaking, there exist two awesomely powerful, almost miraculous, tools that virtually anyone can use: *thinking* and *behaving*. After reading the Action strategies described in Chapter 5, you will have begun to acquire the anti-binge skills and techniques needed to make your thoughts and behaviors work for you.

ATTITUDE   The ultimate goal of the AAA binge-breaking program is not so much loss of weight as loss of self-defeating attitudes and behaviors. Our philosophy is that weight loss and adaptive eating habits will come naturally and easily once you have worked out for yourself a lifestyle you can live with. Just as no pill, potion, or diet plan can stop you from responding to television commercials that dare you to eat only one potato chip or resist a particular brand of cake, so no pill, potion, or diet plan substitute for determination, motivation, and constructive attitude and behavior change. It is only when you get your life under control that your eating will become controllable. It is only when you are ready to acknowledge that you've been using ice cream as consolation that you can appreciate it as a reward. The successful graduate of the AAA binge-breaking program is one who has an awareness of himself and his eating habits and a working knowledge of anti-binge Action strategies. But much more than that, the successful graduate has developed a sense of ease and comfort with himself. Such a person realizes that any positive effects of awareness obtained or actions taken can potentially be as short-lived and temporary as the effects of last year's protein, water, or grapefruit diet; *awareness and action must be accompanied by positive attitude/behavior change and sincere commitment to a new and more adaptive lifestyle.*

In Chapter 6 we will point out that the very idea that such positive change is attainable is very threatening to many bingers. In fact, attitude and behavior change can be so threatening that numerous myths about the process of weight loss have sprung up and become quite popular. Each of these myths is designed to console and reassure bingers that they need never undergo lasting, positive change in their lives. Each of these myths is designed to shift responsibility for faulty eating habits to something vague and intangible like a faulty gene, a faulty gland, or a "disease" called foodaholism. Of course, there are people with eating problems who do have endocrinological or genetic impairments (i.e., "faulty" glands or genes); but these people are in the vast minority of bingers. For most of us, binging is a state of mind, not a state of hunger. And as we shall see in Chapter 6, gaining control of your binging means gaining control of your life in general.

All too many of my weight-problem patients have told me a familiar tale of going up and down not only in weight, but in their very commitment to dieting. Many of these patients have already had years of therapy before coming to see me, and they are quite proficient at verbalizing insights. Intelligent and well-read on the subject of weight loss, many of these patients believe they already have acquired the awareness and action skills necessary to end binging behavior. Why then can't they break the binging habit?

The specific answer to this question varies from patient to patient, but generally speaking, the answer lies in the fact that overeating—in addition to being a reaction to a negative emotional state such as "nervousness" or boredom—may serve some purpose in the binger's life. For example, remaining overweight is helpful for a woman in keeping men at a distance sexually. This distance will be desirable for the woman who is terrified of sexual intercourse and for the happily married woman who unconsciously fears she might be unfaithful to her husband if she slimmed down. I call the moment and process of getting in touch with the *raison d'être* of poor eating and dieting habits as a "Moment of Truth." The Moment of Truth is that momentous turning point in a person's life when the reason he or she has self-destructively binged in the past becomes evident. When this moment of insight into the past is accompanied by unshakable resolve to behave differently in the future—as well as positive change in attitudes and behavior—the urge to binge has been broken for good. At that point, food is robbed of its power to put you out of control, and it no longer represents anything other than food.

Before attempting to reach your Moment of Truth or any goal at all, you must know where you are. As you read Chapter 2, ask yourself, "How many of the twenty-one varieties of binges do I indulge in?" As you read Chapter 3, ask yourself, "How many of these binge games do I play?" The more types you fit into and the more games you play, the more carefully you had better read the rest of this book.

2

The 21 varieties

1. The lone binge

This is one of the most frequent types of binges. It is practiced by single, divorced, and widowed people who perceive themselves as being alone in the world. It also occurs in married people who similarly perceive themselves as alone due to the lack of sufficient attention from their spouses. Lone Bingers are people who prefer to do their binging in solitary. The Lone Binger's relationship with food is an exciting, intimate experience—one not to be shared with (or witnessed by) others. A salad may serve the purpose of having a "living, breathing *something*" to relate to. Lone Bingers also tend to be too embarrassed to eat rich desserts in the company of others, though their freezers are frequently filled with ice cream and other goodies.

Lone Binges are most frequently brought on by conscious or unconscious thoughts similar to: "If I can't have a love affair with a person, I'm going to have one with chocolate chip cookies" or "If no one loves me, I'm going to love myself—with food."

ARE YOU A LONE BINGER?
- Do you binge in solitary?
- Does what you eat in the company of others differ radically from what you would eat when you are entirely on your own?
- Are you at ease with yourself when you are alone for extended periods of time?
- Is food your most faithful companion?
- Have you ever had a "love affair" with chocolate chip cookies?
- Regardless of whether you are married, single, or divorced, do you feel alone in the world?

2. The vengeful binge

The Vengeful Binge is the product of a need to hurt not only yourself, but someone else as well. The Vengeful Binger is one who perceives himself as wronged, slighted, or in some way hurt by another. For example, one woman I saw in therapy described how, for her European-born parents, the "sun rose and set" on her older brother. All of this patient's accomplishments were made light of next to those of her brother. As a result of utter powerlessness and hopelessness with respect to winning her parents' love, this patient rebelled against her mother and father by using Italian sausage and spaghetti as weapons. The patient's anger at her brother for robbing her of parental attention reflected itself in binging that kept her heavy and unattractive to men in general.

The number of reasons for a Vengeful Binge is as legion as the number of Vengeful Bingers. Some more examples of the thinking that consciously or unconsciously goes into a Vengeful Binge are:

"My employer wants me to be thin. . . . Well I'll show him!"

"I'll stay fat as long as my husband (or anyone) isn't going to pay attention to me anyway!"

"I'll make those around me feel guilty about the way they are treating me by cleaning out the refrigerator and then telling them that it's their fault!"

ARE YOU A VENGEFUL BINGER?

· Do you turn to food as a means of hurting yourself or others?

· Do you find yourself to be unable to vent hostility through "normal" channels?

· Do you attempt to elicit guilt in others for your own improper eating?

3. The masquerade binge

This binge occurs in those who are not mentally ready to accept themselves as a thin person after they have lost a significant amount of weight. At a luncheon or elsewhere you may casually inform a new acquaintance that you are watching your weight. The new acquaintance (who did not know you in your fat days) is somewhat surprised and remarks, "My, you don't have a weight problem." You say "Thank you" aloud but secretly think to yourself, "Ha! Little do you know!" You feel as if you have put one over on someone. You feel as if you are in a disguise and that the "thin clothes" you are wearing are a mere costume. You feel all of this because you were not prepared *psychologically* for your weight loss and there remains an "obese brain" in the body of a slim person.

As you eat at the luncheon the terror of being in disguise mounts. What if you are discovered and unmasked for who you really are? Just as Cinderella's coach turned back into a pumpkin at midnight, so you wonder when the masquerade will end and everything will go back to "normal." Believing that it is all a masquerade and that you are really a "foodaholic" leads to anxiety which in turn leads to that old-faithful response—overeating. Within weeks, perhaps months, you have caused your worst fears about the masquerade to come true; you have worked toward fulfilling your own prophecy. Anxiety about masquerading, anxiety about being a so-called foodaholic has led to overeating. And by your own actions you have proved your (unfounded) belief that, for you, being thin is only a masquerade.

ARE YOU A MASQUERADE BINGER?
- Do you think you are fooling others when you lose weight?
- Do you feel you are in disguise in "thin clothes"?
- Are you unwilling to accept yourself slimmed down?

4. The bored binge

Tedious, tiresome, dull, and uninteresting tasks are part of living. Who among us has not had to do dishes, iron shirts, or sort socks? Some people, most visibly those who work on assembly-line-type jobs, earn their living through monotony. And just as each of us must put up with varying amounts of tedium in our daily lives, so we all need breaks from the everyday grind. There are myriad ways to break with routine. For example, you can learn some new isometric exercises, take a walk in a new neighborhood, or take up needlepoint. The much-preferred way to break with routine for the Bored Binger is to become engrossed in eating.

The Bored Binge is an unplanned binge. It happens quite spontaneously when the binger wants to "experience" and "feel" something and finds food the most convenient thing to "experience" and "feel." A patient of mine who had a job interview at 1 P.M. was called at 10 A.M. and asked to come in three hours later than originally planned. She now had all that extra time on her hands and she didn't know what to do with it. As it turned out, she gained not only three extra hours, but about as many pounds as she passed the time whittling at ice cream and cake.

ARE YOU A BORED BINGER?
- Do you turn to food when sorting socks or engaging in other irksome activities?

· When you find yourself with time on your hands is there food in your mouth?
· Is eating what you do to "feel" or "experience" something?

---

5. The "off" binge

"Struggle" is a word that aptly describes many dieters' experiences with trying to lose weight. The trouble is that many dieters believe that they either are struggling or they are not struggling —in other words, it is *all* or *none*; there is no in-between. More specifically, they believe that they are either On or Off their diet. When they are On, nothing in the world can shake their determination. Tempting treats and the most stressful conditions present no problem to the dieter who is On. Unfortunately, it works the opposite way when they are Off. The dieter who construes himself as Off has given himself license to binge. The dieter who is Off can be deprived of nothing, and ice cream, chocolates, and other high-calorie foods are the menu of the day.

Off binging is frequently the result of some deviation, however minor, from a diet. Consider the case of Alma who had been dieting steadily and gradually for weeks with good results. At a restaurant party for a girl friend who was getting divorced, Alma was able to select foods that fit within the caloric goal she had set for herself. However, by the time dessert rolled around Alma's willpower was weakening. She consented to the demand of her girl friend that she taste the creamy French cheesecake. No sooner had Alma tasted it then she construed herself as "Off." Once she believed she was Off, Alma quickly ordered a portion of cheesecake for herself. She also finished some leftover chocolate mousse that another member of the party had rejected. She topped off the evening with corned beef hash under sunnyside-up eggs (with buttered toast) shortly before going to bed. All of this because Alma had become guilt-ridden about going Off and "ruining everything" she had worked for. Alma did not allow herself the rational alternative of believing that she had simply deviated from her diet but was still basically On. It was all somehow easier and more convenient to just throw up her hands and proclaim herself to be Off.

ARE YOU AN "OFF" BINGER?

· Do you think of yourself as being either On or Off a diet with no in-between?
· Do you eat large quantities of high-calorie foods when you see yourself as Off?

---

6. The insecure binge

An Insecure Binge begins with the feeling of inadequacy. This feeling comes from a perceived lack of equality with another individual, most typically a spouse or lover. A wife may be troubled by a self-perception that she is not as intelligent, good looking, witty, etc. as her husband. As these feelings of insecurity mount, they manifest themselves in tension. Compulsive eating serves to quell the aroused state of the body which was caused by this tension. But there is at least one other reason the Insecure Binger is driven to eat: Such a binger may be asking his spouse (or anyone else) to verify that "if you really love me, you'll love me fat."

Chronic Insecure Binging leads to extreme obesity, severe emotional distress, and poor physical health. Life with an Insecure Binger is a trying experience for a spouse. Because the causes of the insecurity frequently lie within the binger's perception of reality rather than in the reality itself, the life of the Insecure Binger's spouse is a life of reassurance and sympathy. As one husband of an Insecure Binger put it, "I feel like I'm walking on eggs while my wife is eating them."

ARE YOU AN INSECURE BINGER?

· Do you believe that someone close to you is somehow "better" than you and does this belief prompt you to eat?
· Do you harbor basic feelings of inadequacy which prompt you to eat?
· Do you believe something is very wrong with you despite sincere assurances from those around you?

---

7. The holiday binge

Christmas, Easter, Mother's Day, Thanksgiving, your birthday—these and other special days are supposed to be joyous occasions. Unfortunately, they are the most miserable times of the year for a good segment of the population. Why is this so? One reason is that we all have different associations to these holidays. If one spent the majority of childhood Christmases in a warm, loving, and generally happy home, Christmas time would be associated with that warmth as an adult. However, if a child grew up in a home where Christmas time was associated with the sight of the parents arguing about money, a relative becoming recklessly drunk, etc., then that person's associations with this period of the year will probably be negative. A Holiday Binge may occur as an attempt to recapture the warmth and nurturance that existed in the childhood home or it may come about as a way of relieving the tension that is associated with a horrible time of year. More food is typically around on holidays, thus facilitating the Holiday Binge.

Some of these special days bring on similar kinds of feelings in many people regardless of their backgrounds. For example, birthdays and New Year's Day are, almost universally, times when many people ask themselves "What have I done with my life? What am I doing now? Where am I going?" These momentous questions almost always raise the state of bodily tension, and the result may be a binge. There are enough holidays the year round to make Holiday Binging a very serious problem to millions of people.

ARE YOU A HOLIDAY BINGER?

· Do you eat significantly more on holidays than you do on other days?
· Do you attempt to recapture the past pleasures of holidays with food?
· Do you attempt to drown the past tensions of holidays with food?

---

8. The wait-until-dark binge

The house is still. Everyone is securely tucked into bed and fast asleep. Suddenly an intruder's step breaks the stillness in the kitchen. The refrigerator door is jerked open; a 40-watt stream of light escapes from the chilly interior; the rye bread is rifled and some cream cheese is violated. A 211 is in progress. This means that it is 2:11 in the morning and a Wait-Until-Dark Binge is about to take place.

The Wait-Until-Dark ("WUD") Binger is usually, though not necessarily, someone who holds a full-time job during the day. A popular *modus operandi* (M.O.) of the WUD Binger is to eat irregularly during the day hours and to make nightly forays into the kitchen. However, the M.O. may vary as a function of the marital status of the WUD, the amount of policing there is of the kitchen by concerned family members, and the penalties (if any) imposed for sneak-thiefing. Rehabilitation for the WUD Binger frequently entails the prescription of more regular daily (and day-ly) eating habits and religious adherence to the Awareness and Action strategies described in Chapters 4 and 5.

ARE YOU A "WUD" BINGER?
- Are you too busy during the day to think about food?
- Do you experience hunger in dim light?
- Have you ever felt like a "sneak thief" in the kitchen?

---

9. The out-of-the-blues binge

Also called the Depressed Binge, this is probably one of the most prevalent types of binges in American society. It occurs when, for any number of reasons, you are feeling "blue" or depressed and you turn to the freezer as your therapist. Like the Vengeful Binge, this type of binge may actually be prompted by anger. However, it is a different kind of anger—*an anger turned against the self*. Whereas the Vengeful Binger is eating to hurt others, the Blue Binger usually is eating to comfort himself. Often such a binger has a feeling of helplessness with regard to the events taking place around him, but in eating they are in control (even though they are really out of control). Meals and snacks sometimes serve the purpose of being the only "palatable" moments for the Blue Binger to reflect on how cruel the world can be. When Blue Bingers do not have their time occupied with binging, they spend much of it resting, lazily watching television, or sleeping. Because they feel so down, they find it very difficult to give their all to anyone or anything—except food.

ARE YOU A BLUE BINGER?
- Do you turn to food when you are depressed, blue, or broken-hearted?
- Are you one of those who turn anger inward and eat as a result?
- Do you feel helpless about certain events that are happening around you and do you console yourself with food?

· Do you find yourself sleeping much more than you want to, eating much more than you have to, and generally doing less of the things you'd like to be doing?

---

10. The long-distance binge

Food is a natural complement to travel. Most of us look forward to sampling the local fare when we are off to some new place. But half the fun is getting there.

One of the main reasons eating and overeating are such reliable traveling companions is related to those equally reliable states—anxiety and tension—which frequently accompany travelers from the time of their departure to their return. There is usually the element of the unknown and the unexpected when we travel, and this can be both exciting and disconcerting. No matter how planned the itinerary might be, there are always questions concerning what lies ahead. Similarly, anxiety and tension may be generated by thoughts of all the things waiting for you when you return. There may also be anxiety related to your thoughts about the mode of transportation you are using, whether it be air, land, or sea.

Some people handle travel anxiety the same way they deal with other uncomfortable bodily states—they turn to food. And food is readily available on most forms of transportation. The airlines have learned well the value of inflight food and drink, and the steamship companies have made elaborate gourmet cuisine one of the major selling points of their cruise trips. The "club car" is not only a standard part of a train traveling long distances, but it is frequently seen in small commuter lines as well. We all need to eat while traveling long distances, and each of us has probably partaken of meals or snacks aboard trains, boats, and planes. The Long-Distance Binger is the one who overindulges to such a point, that by the end of the journey he is usually ready to "abandon ship."

ARE YOU A LONG-DISTANCE BINGER?

· Is food the first word that comes to your mind when you think of travel?

· Do you overindulge yourself aboard trains, boats, and planes?

---

11. The flirtation-palpitation binge

Also known as the Gentleman's-Attention Binge, this type of overeating pattern occurs most frequently in women who have lost a significant amount of weight and binge as a result of increased male attention. The following consequences of looking good have the power to prompt a Flirtation-Palpitation Binge:

The opposite sex is giving you a lot of attention which you simultaneously like and dislike. You like wearing the clothes and getting all of the flattering attention, but you are genuinely frightened by the sexual overtures and advances the men around you appear to be making. You really don't know how to handle the men and are beginning to become unsure whether you want to bother.

The opposite sex is giving you a lot of attention which you are basking in. You feel sexy when you are thin. In fact, you feel as if your sexual impulses are going haywire. But now you have a new problem: Protecting yourself from a fear of becoming promiscuous. If you are married you may be asking yourself how you will protect yourself from an extramarital affair. When you start asking yourself if being thin is really worth such problems, a Flirtation-Palpitation Binge may result.

You have had platonic, nonsexual relations with a number of people of the opposite sex. Now that you have lost weight you find you are losing all of these spiritual friends because the relationships have become more physical, more sexual, and hence more threatening.

ARE YOU A FLIRTATION-PALPITATION BINGER?

· After you lose weight, are you afraid of attention from the opposite sex and does this fear drive you to binge?
· Do you feel it is "safe" to have friends of the opposite sex only when you are overweight?

---

12. The no-competition binge

Some people appear to thrive on competition and can't get enough of it. Others shun competition and simply drop out if it's at all possible to do so. A No-Competition Binge is a method used for avoiding all of the sources of life's everyday competitions. By engaging in enough of these binges, the binger will become and remain obese and probably use the obesity as a means of dropping out. Obesity is useful in eliminating competition in the job market; all other things being equal, obese people are hired last. If the No-Competition Binger has not dropped out of the job market and is gainfully employed, he or she need not worry about competing in the office in terms of clothes. Obese men will wear anything that fits and obese women need only a wardrobe of a few dark tents. There will also be no competition with regard to the usual intraoffice flirtations—the binger has successfully managed to avoid stirring anyone's imagination. A sufficient number of No-Competition Binges also ensures that you will not have to compete in terms of your personality either. Being obese, you can resign yourself to the fact that people are only going to judge you by what you look like and not what you say. And most importantly, you will not have to compete socially. You'll probably wind up marrying another No-Competition Binger and live happily ever after eradicating competition with calories.

ARE YOU A NO-COMPETITION BINGER?
- Do you shield yourself from competition with your weight?
- Is the thought of competing for a job or for a spouse threatening to you?
- If you lost weight, would you be frightened occupationally or socially?

---

13. The substitute binge

The Substitute Binge is a direct result of some sort of deprivation. Most frequently it is the result of deprivation of a loved one's attention. Unlike the Lone Binge (which may or may not be consciously motivated), the Substitute Binge is almost always a product of conscious choice. The Substitute Binger may not want to get close to people, or he may lack the social skills for doing so. And while the Lone Binger prefers to do his binging in solitary, the Substitute Binger doesn't mind the presence of others. In fact, it is the presence of others (and the presence of deep emotional attachments) that the Substitute Binger is starved for, though he may deny it.

Nurturance from food as a substitute for the nurturance of compassionate, loving, warm, and sensitive human contact is an all-too-frequent phenomenon. As children most of us were exposed to the pairing of food with love and attention. Maribel, a patient of mine who had a penchant for soft, creamy, "baby-type food," binged on such foods as ice cream, farina, and sour cream during times of stress. Maribel remembered vividly how her mother would lovingly spoon-feed her such foods when she was ill and kept home from school. Adults who were institutionalized as children should, in theory, be particularly prone to Substitute Binging. This is so because in many orphanages and other institutions the only time the infants and babies received extended periods of attentive cuddling and holding was during feeding time.

Many people wrongly equate Substitute Binging with insufficient amounts of sexual intercourse. Although this may be true in some cases, clinical experience has shown me that it is not really sex per se which is lacking, but an *emotional* closeness with another individual. Men who frequent prostitutes may feel fulfilled in a physical sense, but seldom do they feel fulfilled in an emotional sense. Similarly, many wives can get all of the physical contact they want from their husbands but remain tragically unfulfilled in terms of a deep emotional experience.

ARE YOU A SUBSTITUTE BINGER?

· Do you substitute your inability to get close to people by getting close to food?
· When it comes to deep emotional relationships do you say, "I'd rather eat than be bothered"?
· When it comes to satisfying interpersonal relationships, are you getting yours?

14. The merry-go-round binge

Are you extra careful about what you eat in public? Or are you the opposite . . . one of those people who acts as if he needs to show the world how much he enjoys overeating? The latter behavior characterizes the Merry-Go-Round Binger. This binger's mission in life may be summed up by the message in some commercials: Since you only go-around once in life, make it a merry go-round. In line with this philosophy, these bingers make an art of showing other people how hard they will work to keep fat on. They seldom deny themselves triple sundaes or double portions of cheesecake.

The tension and underlying problems that prompt a Merry-Go-Round Binge are often denied, concealed, or, at best, made light of. Further, such bingers seldom admit that their eating habits are making them depressed and not merry at all. These bingers are quick to downplay the validity of insurance-company statistics on death and disease rates in obese individuals which indicate that people (particularly men) who take the "go-around once" attitude with respect to food, have an all-too-short go-around.

ARE YOU A MERRY-GO-ROUND BINGER?

- Do you believe that since you "only go-around once" you should make it a merry-go-round with respect to food?
- Do you make light of, deny, or conceal the problems and tensions that cause you to binge?
- Are you unwilling to admit that overeating makes you sad and not merry?

---

15. The extraordinary binge

Any change in routine can occasion a binge in some people. If you are an Extraordinary Binger, you might binge if:

- You get a raise.
- You get fired.
- Your hours at work are changed.
- Your spouse is late from work.
- Your spouse is early from work.
- Your spouse doesn't come home from work.
- Your Aunt Mildred drops in for coffee.
- A fuse blows.
- There is a sudden change in weather.

· You get a flat tire.
· Your favorite television show is pre-empted.
· Your hair dryer malfunctions.
· A houseplant dies.
· You win the lottery.
· A relative gives birth.
· You buy a new car.
· Your daughter gets evicted and decides to move back in with you.

When something out-of-the-ordinary happens, most people attempt to stabilize their life with some sort of "equalizer." For the Extraordinary Binger, that equalizer tends to be their most stable of staples.

ARE YOU AN EXTRAORDINARY BINGER?

· Does a change in routine usually lead you to a craving to eat?
· Do you use food as an "equalizer"?

---

16. The left-out binge

If you have ever had a problem with food you can readily identify with the Left-Out Binge. It happens after you've enviously sat there and watched some thin, "normal" people eating heartily. As you stare at your black coffee, cottage cheese, and lettuce you begin to feel not only deprived but totally "left out" when it comes to the joy of food and the joy of living. Your mind races to the time you were out to lunch with a group of your coworkers or in a restaurant with your family. The waiter asked if you would like dessert and your mind wildly proclaimed "*Yes!*" but your mouth timidly said, "No, not for me, thank you." Some time after these memories leave and the feelings of being deprived, abnormal, and different have had a chance to do their work, you begin a Left-Out Binge. With each bite the Left-Out Binger seems to be proclaiming his commonality with the human race. With each bite the Left-Out Binger seems to be announcing, "I will not be deprived! I will not be different! I will not be left out!" Unfortunately, after the binge the binger still feels left out—only more so.

ARE YOU A LEFT-OUT BINGER?

· Do you feel left out or deprived in restaurants, at barbecues, or in other social eating situations?
· Do you envy thin, "normal" people and do these feelings make food more appealing?
· Are you plagued by feelings of deprivation which can only be relieved by food?

17. The reader's binge

Remember the story of Pavlov? How the repeated pairing of a bell with the presentation of food got dogs to salivate at the sound of the bell? Think about Pavlov's dogs as you read about the Reader's Binge—and put down anything you're eating!

A Reader's Binge is one of those binges which usually occur before the reader has a chance to realize what has happened. Reading Binges occur in people who, for long periods of time, have paired reading with eating. One reader I treated was a college student named Marge. According to Marge, her life revolved around studying and food. Marge tried to spend every available moment reading and/or eating—when she wasn't sleeping. Marge read in the campus library, by the lake, in bed just before going to sleep, and, of most interest to us, while eating breakfast, lunch, and dinner.

One of the questions I asked Marge at the time of her initial visit to my office was, "How many meals per day do you usually eat?" After a moment of reflection Marge smiled impishly and replied, "One." This answer revealed Marge's insights into her problem eating habits. As a result of the constant pairing of eating with reading, Marge had conditioned herself to salivate at the sight of her books. The resulting habit involved non-verbalized thoughts such as "If I'm reading therefore I must be hungry." If this sounds strange to you, remember that Pavlov's dogs heard the bell ringing and "thought" they were hungry (as evidenced by the flow of saliva). Consistent pairing of eating with responses other than reading such as watching television may also come to elicit salivation.

ARE YOU A READING BINGER?
- Do you pair reading with eating?
- Do you salivate at the sight of books?
- Do you gain weight every time you finish a book?

---

18. The size-up binge

Many of my overweight patients have reported that they feel as if they are being "sized-up" when they walk into a room. The person doing the sizing-up may be as close to the patient as her mother or a total stranger. The sizing-up process not only takes into account your figure, but everything else about you that you may feel is inadequate, such as your hair, your skin, and your make-up. The Size-Up Binge occurs after the evaluation you think you have flunked.

Size-Up Bingers live by other people's standards and are notorious for looking at themselves through other people's eyes. Interestingly, a second party need not even be in the room for a Size-Up Binge to take place. For one of my patients, just the thought of her mother looking disapprovingly at her body was enough to spur Size-Up Binging. She felt that she had let her mother down by letting herself go. The predictable result of the Size-Up Binge is going up one size when it is over.

ARE YOU A SIZE-UP BINGER?

· Does the feeling that you are being evaluated by someone prompt you to binge?
· Do you go up a clothing size after a family reunion?
· Are you living your life through other people's eyes with other people's standards?

---

19. The worry binge

Also known as the Wary Binge, but not to be confused with the Weary Binge (number 20), the Worry Binge is employed by people who use food as a tranquilizer. We have all run into Worried Bingers. You know, the people who sit with glazed donuts until they have glazed eyes. They always seem to be worried about something, and they use food to numb the brain, dull the senses, and ease the pain. A patient of mine whose husband was a fireman in New York City found herself Worry Binging if her husband was as little as half an hour late coming home from work. Despite the fact that she ate herself into a stupor, she still would not forget why she was worrying. The horrible thing about a Worry Binge is that it gives the binger a lot more to worry about when it is over.

My patient's Worry Binging ended when she found another activity with which to occupy herself while worrying about her husband's safety. She would clean out her closets and drawers until he came home. People who make Worry Binging a lifelong habit must, unfortunately, resign themselves to being obese. There are too many things in life to worry about. Simply stated, if you're going to eat every time you're worried about something, you can't afford to worry about overeating.

ARE YOU A WORRY BINGER?

- Is food your tranquilizer when you are anxious?
- Have you ever eaten to the point of numbness?
- Do you try to escape from problems by "losing yourself" in food?

---

20. The weary binge

This type of gorging behavior frequently occurs within ten minutes after coming home from work. The hallmark of Weary Binging is a sense of being mentally drained and physically fatigued combined with the belief that, somehow, a large quantity of food will restore a feeling of freshness. A patient of mine who worked on the floor of the New York Stock Exchange regularly engaged in Weary Binges. Frazzled from the day's frantic activities, he would experience a "let down" and a feeling of exhaustion by the time he made it home. Routinely he would scavenge the refrigerator searching for something to perk him up. It wasn't until this patient learned to discriminate hunger from weariness that he learned to lie down when feeling let down.

ARE YOU A WEARY BINGER?

- Does your refrigerator door open within ten minutes after you come home from work?
- Do you use food to perk you up when you are exhausted?
- Do you confuse feelings of weariness with feelings of hunger?

21. The renaissance binge

You've just lost a substantial amount of weight and you look great. You feel great. You're light on your feet, you're being noticed, and you feel like a "new you" in many respects. Amidst all your mental celebration there is a longing—perhaps it is an unconscious longing—for the simple, uncomplicated days when you were heavy. You know . . . those days when you didn't have to shop for hours for clothes and any dark-colored tent was alright. You remember . . . those days when you didn't have to worry about attention from the opposite sex and you could be totally preoccupied with yourself. Is it all coming back to you?

As you stare into your clothes closet and gaze at all your "fat clothes," a moment of hesitation comes over you. You want to take them and throw them away forever but something is stopping you. You are unsure. You start to wonder what you will have to wear should you get fat again and then you scold yourself for even thinking like that. As the tension and anxiety stemming from your ambivalence builds, you being to experience that old feeling of hunger that isn't really hunger. A binge that is the direct result of your success in achieving a "new you"—a Renaissance Binge—is about to occur. Should Renaissance Binging persist over an extended period of time, the problem of what to do about the old clothes will be solved.

ARE YOU A RENAISSANCE BINGER?

· Does a substantial amount of weight loss prompt you to binge?
· When and if you have reached the "new you" you have wanted, have you been complacent and satisfied, or disappointed and disillusioned with your life?

Binge games . . .

3

You lose when

you win!

A wealth of clinical experience with weight patients has shown me that game playing with diets and weight-loss programs is quite common. Are you a diet-game player? Is self-destruction one of your missions in life? Do you enjoy frequent binging while telling others that you are trying to lose weight? If so, the following binge games are likely to be all too familiar to you.

On the other hand you may be someone who has truly had enough of binge games. You may have reached a stage in your life when you are genuinely willing to experiment with constructive, lifesaving anti-binge-game strategies. If that is the case, the Awareness and Action games described in Chapters 4 and 5 will be of greater relevance to you in terms of the way you presently live or want to live. But Awareness and Action are only two of the three components in the AAA program of binge-breaking. The third and final component, Attitude, is discussed in Chapter 6. This is where all of the game playing ends and a constructive, more adaptive lifestyle begins.

For now, regardless of what stage you are at in your personal binge-breaking program, it will be helpful for you to carefully read the following binge game descriptions. Read them with an eye toward prevention. For the sake of your health, your looks, and the welfare of those who love and depend on you, guard against ever playing any of these games again.

Hide 'n' sneak

OBJECT OF THE GAME   To successfully hide and then sneak-eat the largest quantity of food.

HOW THE GAME IS PLAYED   This is a game for a binger who is married or living with a concerned partner. The idea is to trick the partner into believing that you are not deviating from some prescribed diet. Actually, you are bringing home all kinds of cakes, cookies, and other empty-calorie foods and successfully hiding them all over the house for some future binge. This game can be played by any number of bingers, and the one who gains the most weight over a specified period of time is declared the winner.

Sweet monopoly

OBJECT OF THE GAME   To eat every last sweet thing in the house.

HOW THE GAME IS PLAYED   This game is most exciting when played by bingers who are members of large families. The binger's goal is to have consumed every sweet thing around before anyone else has realized what has happened. The play begins on Wednesday evening or whenever the family food shopping for the week is done. Bingers who have no business playing this game (i.e., those who have diabetes, heart trouble, or related conditions) must take a Chance card after every bite.

Russian-dressing roulette

OBJECT OF THE GAME   To avoid getting caught with the empty salad-dressing server.

HOW THE GAME IS PLAYED   The play begins at lunchtime when a group of six bingers order salads and diet salad dressing in a restaurant. After the waiter informs the group that the restaurant does not carry any diet dressings (something that everyone knew anyway), the boldest binger in the group orders Russian dressing. At this point all of the other players resolve to eat their salads dry. The orders are brought and the boldest one goes first, shooting the dressing onto every side of the assorted vegetables. One by one the other players become excited by the sight and smell of the Russian dressing, and they ask that it be passed to them. No one knows when their luck or the dressing is going to run out. The loser of this game is the player who is holding the server when it runs out of dressing. He or she must pick up the check and leave the tip.

Pick-up sticks

OBJECT OF THE GAME   To scoop up as many pretzel sticks as possible with two hands.

HOW THE GAME IS PLAYED   A popular game at social gatherings where copious quantities of pretzel sticks are freely available, this game can be played by two or more players. All that is needed in the way of equipment is one oversized punch bowl filled to the brim with pretzel sticks. Bingers line up and one by one scoop out as many pretzels as they can handle with two hands. The winner is determined by the pretzel count or weight. Broken pretzels and those that have fallen on the floor don't count. All participants must eat all the pretzels they have scooped. This game can also be played with potato or corn chips, in which case it is called Pick-Up Chips.

Giant steps

OBJECT OF THE GAME   To take the greatest number of giant steps both forward and back.

HOW THE GAME IS PLAYED   This is a game that is based on the hard-core bingers' philosophy that any growth or progress in losing and keeping off unwanted pounds must be accompanied by regression to a more unsatisfactory state of affairs. The play begins when a binger believes he has finally begun to obtain some control over his problem eating habits. This "giant step" in his life may have been responsible for the loss of, say, ten pounds. But now, if the binger is to be successful at this game, he must quickly gain ten pounds. Any number of bingers can play, and the winner is the one who has taken the most giant steps forward and back.

Boston marathon

OBJECT OF THE GAME   To eat Boston cream pie until you can't.

HOW THE GAME IS PLAYED   Sheer endurance is the key to winning this binge game. Bingers who have played it before know the value of pacing themselves from start to finish and of proper breathing and mental attitude. This marathon is not timed. The winner is the binger who has completely devoured the greatest number of Boston cream pies. In case of tie, a runoff is held using baked Alaska.

Indianapolis 500

OBJECT OF THE GAME   To eat the most snacks per week that are 500 calories or more.

HOW THE GAME IS PLAYED   Inspired by the famous auto race, this Indy 500 is a race for calories. The idea is, every time you sit down to eat, think about what snack you can have later that will be at least 500 or more calories. All bingers participating in this game are responsible for keeping accurate accounts of not only the number of snacks they've had, but the total number of calories of each snack. In case of a tie for the greatest number of snacks, the winner is determined by the highest calorie count. Prizes usually include steel-belted radial tires to wear to the beach.

Championship weightlifting

OBJECT OF THE GAME   To gain the most number of pounds within one eight-hour period.

HOW THE GAME IS PLAYED   Bingers who participate in this game are usually those who approach the sport with a great deal of practice, training, and discipline in nonstop eating. Since each participant has only eight hours to raise their weight by the maximum number of pounds, selection of foods that are highest in calories is crucial. Veteran competitors are those who have learned to minimize their arm and mouth movements while eating so that calories will not be wasted on expenditures of energy. All participants are carefully weighed before the competition begins. At the conclusion of the eight-hour period, the participants are again asked to get on the scale (or they are carried to the scale). The person who has lifted his weight the most is declared the winner.

Basket-ball

OBJECT OF THE GAME   To have a ball binging while shopping in a supermarket.

HOW THE GAME IS PLAYED   Bingers are provided with empty shopping baskets to wheel around their favorite supermarket and stuff with high-calorie treats. Bingers must open at least three packages of such treats and completely finish the contents thereof while shopping from a prepared list of groceries. The binger who consumes the greatest number of calories while shopping wins. All foods consumed must come from the binger's own shopping basket, and the calories from foods coming from open packages on the shelves will be declared illegal and disqualified.

Snackgammon

OBJECT OF THE GAME   To use all chance meetings with friends as opportunities to binge.

HOW THE GAME IS PLAYED   Like backgammon, snackgammon is a game of both chance and skill. The play begins when an unexpected guest—a neighbor, a friend, a relative, etc.—suddenly drops in to say hello. The binger must now skillfully prepare coffee and cake to make the snacks irresistible. A snackgammon occurs if the guest drinks the coffee but leaves the cake for the binger. A double-snackgammon occurs if the binger prepares enough food for two or more guests and no one but the binger is hungry.

Football widow

OBJECT OF THE GAME   To consume the greatest number of calories on a Sunday afternoon while your husband is absorbed in football games.

HOW THE GAME IS PLAYED   The opening kickoff of the first televised football game on a Sunday afternoon signals the start of this game. This is traditionally a game for married, female bingers though it may be played by both sexes. The idea here is to engage in nonstop eating while simultaneously thinking to yourself, "He's more interested in football than he is in me!" The rules are: if you have any questions for your husband, you are only allowed to ask them during a commercial—you'll receive an answer during the next commercial. Two-minute warnings are given just prior to the end of each quarter, and half-times are reserved for arguments which are not refereed. The play ends when the clock runs out on the very last game of the afternoon or evening. Bingers who gain twenty pounds or more over the course of a football season qualify as finalists in the last competition of the year: The Super Bowl.

Gin dummy

OBJECT OF THE GAME   To drink as much as you can for the sole purpose of being sociable.

HOW THE GAME IS PLAYED   This is a game played by non-drinkers who wind up binging on gin and tonic or other mixed drinks just to be sociable. This game could begin at a business lunch, at a party, or any other setting in which there is social pressure to drink. Although the nondrinker doesn't even enjoy liquor, he orders a gin and tonic "to be sociable." Subsequently he orders more of the same for the same reason. At the end of the evening the nondrinker who has consumed the most liquor despite the fact that he doesn't even enjoy liquor is crowned "Gin Dummy" and given black coffee and a lift home.

Pokered marshmallows

OBJECT OF THE GAME   To consume more toasted marshmallows than anyone else.

Binge games . . . you lose when you win!

HOW THE GAME IS PLAYED   Pokers or spears are distributed to four to six bingers sitting around a campfire. A wheelbarrow of marshmallows is placed alongside the fire. When the signal is given, bingers must spear, toast, and eat as many marshmallows as they can until the supply is exhausted. Ice water is readily available to all of the participants who will inevitably burn their lips and tongues trying to stuff the marshmallows in. The binger who has speared, toasted, and consumed the greatest number of marshmallows is the winner.

Solitare

OBJECT OF THE GAME   To play games with yourself for an entire evening.

HOW THE GAME IS PLAYED   The play begins when the binger construes himself as "depressed," "blue," "broken-hearted," etc. and then proceeds to allow this mood to act as an excuse for undisciplined gorging of food. During this period the binger may be saying to him- or herself silly things like, "No one needs me anyway" or "My children don't care about me so why should I?" During this game all contact with loved ones who could rationally disprove such nonsense is carefully avoided. A popular game among the frustrated, the depressed, and the emotionally needy, this game is also referred to as Slow Suicide.

Clean plate club

OBJECT OF THE GAME   To gain the most weight over an agreed upon period of time by finishing everything that is on your plate—and on everyone else's as well.

HOW THE GAME IS PLAYED   All that is needed to win this game is some exceptionally large plates which players will want to use for breakfast, lunch, dinner, and in-between-meal treats. Be sure to fill the plate to the brim; if you go for seconds the rule is you must fill the plate to the brim again. Winners of this binge game tend to have exceptional visual-motor abilities but poor language skills. That is, while they may be able to move food quickly from a plate to their mouth, they may have difficulty understanding the meaning of certain words—such as "leftovers."

Trampoline

OBJECT OF THE GAME   To bounce up and down, as high as possible, in commitment to sensible eating habits.

HOW THE GAME IS PLAYED   Players begin by having only black coffee in the morning and black coffee with diet cottage cheese for lunch. Some time before dinner the binger says to himself, "Well, all I had for breakfast was black coffee and all I had for lunch was black coffee and cottage cheese, so I'm entitled to something before dinner." Players then snack on various crackers and nuts before dinner and indulge themselves freely in food if they are involved in preparing dinner. By the time dinner is served the player does not feel very hungry and eats an extremely small portion. Some time after dinner each binger then says to himself, "Well, all I had for breakfast was black coffee and all I had for lunch was black coffee and cottage cheese, and I didn't have very much dinner, so therefore I'm entitled to something." Players then proceed to finish a pound of chocolate-covered graham crackers and half a quart of skimmed milk. At this point the game for that day ends and all of the players go to bed.

Pantry raid

OBJECT OF THE GAME   To plan and successfully stage a raid on a hostess's pantry.

HOW THE GAME IS PLAYED   The play begins when the binger is invited to be an overnight guest in the home of a friend, relative, or acquaintance. Players then have from the time the lights go out until sunrise to raid the hostess's pantry and consume as much as possible without being discovered. If it is an exceptionally large house and there are two pantries, players may earn double points by successfully getting in and out of both of them.

Arm wrestling

OBJECT OF THE GAME   To out-binge your opponent by wrestling food away from the concerned family members.

HOW THE GAME IS PLAYED   Only bingers with concerned family members may play. The play begins when a binger takes a half gallon of ice cream out of the refrigerator fully intent on finishing it off (other foods can be substituted). After the wrapping has been torn asunder and the first spoonfuls drawn, a concerned family member who has discovered what is happening attempts to physically remove the food from the binger. This is where the test of strength begins. Bingers receive five points if they can successfully wrestle the ice cream away from their concerned family member and then go on to finish it. However, bingers can receive an extra five-point bonus if they can get their concerned family member to utter the words, "Go ahead and eat it—you're only killing yourself and I won't try to stop you again!" The binger who has accumulated the most points within a given time period wins.

Eating for strength

OBJECT OF THE GAME   To consume the largest quantity of food in one sitting under the guise of "eating for strength."

HOW THE GAME IS PLAYED   The play begins when the binger complains of some vague pain, most typically a headache. The binger does not feel particularly hungry but thinks that eating may somehow relieve the pain. The result is a spur-of-the-moment binge that not only fails to relieve the pain but adds depression and guilt as a result. This game is popular in a variety of situations where food has been equated with strength. Persons who feel ill, persons who indulge in any kind of sport or physical activity, and persons who indulge in inordinate amounts of sexual activity may all feel that they must eat large quantities of food to "keep their strength up."

Dog racing

OBJECT OF THE GAME   To eat as many hot dogs as possible in a thirty-minute sitting.

HOW THE GAME IS PLAYED   All bingers have their favorite hot dog places. In this game the habit of overeating hot dogs is now worth valuable points. Give yourself three points for every hot dog eaten plain and five points for every one eaten with the roll. Mustard, sauerkraut, onions, and other toppings will get you another two points. You may have french fried potatoes and a drink, but these foods will not figure into your total number of binge points. The winner is the person who has scored the most points within one thirty-minute sitting, and the prize is a one-year supply of buns.

Pin the tail on the tailor

OBJECT OF THE GAME   To recite the greatest number of expletives to the tailor for ruining your clothes even though he is not at fault.

HOW THE GAME IS PLAYED   The play begins sometime after a recent binge as the binger is trying on some clothes returned from the tailor. The clothes do not fit properly and the binger is steamed. The binger calls the tailor to give him a piece of his mind. The binger is allowed a maximum phone connection time of three minutes to utter as many expletives as he can before the tailor tells him that it is the binger's fluctuations in weight that are responsible for the poor fit of his clothes.

Fruits of my labor

OBJECT OF THE GAME   To eat the most food while preparing dinner, baking a cake, etc.

HOW THE GAME IS PLAYED   Bingers playing this game must be prepared to sip while measuring, taste while slicing, and nibble while chopping. This is a food-preparation game designed to allow the binger to binge in the name of "quality control." This game is a favorite among binging cooks who look forward to tasting batters and other rich concoctions "without going off the diet." Of course when the final product is ready—whether it is a full course dinner, a chocolate fudge cake, peanut butter cookies, or whatever—the binger must taste the fruit of his or her labor. The binger who consumes the greatest number of calories from all stages of the food-preparation project wins.

Till . . .

OBJECT OF THE GAME   To come up with the most creative excuse for a binge.

HOW THE GAME IS PLAYED   Bingers must finish the following sentence in twenty-five words or less: I was "good" until . . .

. . . .
. . . .

Enter as often as you wish, but remember that each entry must be accompanied by the side panel of your favorite box of cookies. Entries will be judged on the basis of their originality, appropriateness, and their ability to place responsibility for the binge off you and onto something else. First prize could be an all-expense-paid, three-year trip to law school.

Brains not body

OBJECT OF THE GAME   To binge so that people will appreciate you for your brains, not your body.

HOW THE GAME IS PLAYED   This game usually begins when a freakish event happens: an overweight, female binger is complimented on her body by the milkman or someone else who holds a relatively unimportant place in her life. The compliment trips the binge mechanism in the brain which has long ago resolved that men will have to love her for her brains, not her body. And so, like many of the other binge games, the idea here is to gain the maximum amount of weight in the minimum amount of time.

No choice

OBJECT OF THE GAME To structure your environment in such a way that you always have "no choice" when it comes to problem foods.

HOW THE GAME IS PLAYED The play begins when the binger declares himself to be on a diet. He then proceeds to allow himself to deviate from the diet whenever he has "no choice" but to eat problem foods. The idea is to schedule as many "no choice" situations as you can in a one-week period. For some players such a situation might be a business luncheon complete with alcoholic beverages and a full course meal, a trip to Grandma Zelda's, or a day at the county fair. The winner is the binger who structures his environment in such a way that he is in a "no choice" situation at least once a day.

Commercial vehicle

OBJECT OF THE GAME To eat as much as possible during one station break.

HOW THE GAME IS PLAYED This game is usually played at or about 8:30 P.M. The binger has been watching some prime-time television program when suddenly a series of commercials designed to foster compulsive eating and binging bombard him. The viewer is dared into compulsive eating by commercials that tell him that "nobody can eat just one" potato chip and "nobody can resist" a brand of cake. In this game, letting the commercials propel you into the kitchen is a deliberate, not an unconscious, phenomenon. The binger who gains the most weight during one station break wins a one-year supply of TV dinners.

Coffee and . . .

OBJECT OF THE GAME   To go out for coffee with a friend and wind up having coffee and. . . .

HOW THE GAME IS PLAYED   Two bingers go out to a local coffee shop. Their primary purpose is to satisfy their need for conversation, not their need for food. Their intention is to have a cup of coffee and some good conversation. Once in the coffee shop that good intention becomes blurred as the sight and smells of the food massage the senses. By the time the waiter comes over and asks, "Are you ready to order?" the two bingers are *really* ready. And what was once a desire for a cup of coffee and some good conversation has now become a desire for a cup of coffee and some good cheese danish. The binger who takes in the greatest number of calories wins.

If I'm in the kitchen, I must be hungry

OBJECT OF THE GAME   To binge simply because you are in the kitchen.

HOW THE GAME IS PLAYED   The play begins any time after dinner when a player finds himself in the kitchen. He may be in the kitchen because he is doing the dishes, because he is searching for something, because he is passing to another room —virtually any reason will do. Once in the kitchen, the player's right hand is drawn to the refrigerator-door handle out of sheer force of habit. Something in the refrigerator catches the binger's eye and it is instantly consumed. Skilled players should be able to concoct myriad excuses for being in the kitchen at all hours of the day and night. Players get ten points for all food eaten out of force of habit alone and five points for all food they actually taste and enjoy.

Ending it all

OBJECT OF THE GAME   To finish every fattening food in the house before beginning a new diet.

HOW THE GAME IS PLAYED   The play begins when the binger resolves to seriously begin to diet. The only obstacle standing in the way of this latest effort is that bag of potato chips and that box of donuts that must still somehow be disposed of. Players reason that if they just finish all "taboo" foods remaining around the house (i.e., if they "end it all") they will be ready to begin the diet of their lifetime. Immediately players begin taking the first important steps to weight loss by completely finishing the potato chips and the donuts. The winner at this game is the binger who puts on the most weight prior to beginning a diet.

Slack off

OBJECT OF THE GAME   To slack off in progress as much as possible after you begin to obtain control over problem eating habits.

HOW THE GAME IS PLAYED   This is a game in which the unconscious command to "slack off" is given to a dieter at some crucial point in a weight-control program. Exactly why the message is given will vary with the unique needs and life situations of the individual dieters. We will have more to say about slacking off in Chapter 6 when we discuss the Moment of Truth concept. Here it will simply be pointed out that the winner of this game is the dieter who has shown by virtue of his or her binges that he has slacked off the most and is back to ground zero both in weight control and in mental attitude toward food.

Good neighbor policy

OBJECT OF THE GAME   To eat as much as possible at your neighbor's house.

HOW THE GAME IS PLAYED   Many bingers make an honest effort—or so they think—not to binge. They think they are helping themselves, for example, by keeping problem foods out of their house. The difficulty of course is that problem foods can be found anywhere, even right next door. This game is played by consuming large quantities of such problem foods while commiserating with your next-door neighbor and swearing not to bring those foods into *your* house. In some cases, bingers have reported that they have the key to their neighbor's house for emergency reasons and have used that key to go in and munch on cookies and candies they do not keep in their own house.

I will if you will

OBJECT OF THE GAME   To binge wildly because a fellow dieter has agreed to binge right alongside of you.

HOW THE GAME IS PLAYED   This is a game based on the philosophy that there is safety in numbers. The safety referred to is safety from gaining weight. The calories taken in will somehow be nullified—or the pain will somehow be lessened— if a fellow binger decides to deviate with you. This game is over when the binger realistically decides there is no such safety in numbers and the philosophy guiding his or her behavior really has been "misery loves company."

Midtown distressway

OBJECT OF THE GAME   To thoroughly gorge oneself with food after a bout with heavy traffic.

HOW THE GAME IS PLAYED   After a miserable hour or two or three in horrible traffic the player decides that he must reward himself with a treat. One or two or three hours later, after the player has sufficiently rewarded himself, he computes the number of calories he has consumed. If the number of calories the player expended while sitting in traffic is equal to one percent of the number of calories contained in the food consumed, the player wins. However, the player loses if the number of calories expended in traffic was less than one percent of the total amount taken in on the binge. Most players lose this game.

Beautiful binger

OBJECT OF THE GAME   To please your weird husband by binging.

HOW THE GAME IS PLAYED   This game is for female bingers who are married to men who prefer their women heavy and who do everything they can to keep their wives obese. Such husbands are perennially bringing home tempting treats and high-calorie foods. Many wives play right into their husbands hands by eating all of the junk that is brought into the house. These women may not realize that their husbands want them to stay fat to keep them in a "one down" position or that their fat may be gratifying hubby's need to keep his wife unattractive to all other men. Still, women who engage in Beautiful Binging seem to be content with just winning their husband's approval and attention as a prize.

Churn! Churn! Churn!

OBJECT OF THE GAME   To keep your stomach churning for as long as possible.

HOW THE GAME IS PLAYED   "To everything there is a seasoning. . . ." With these words, uttered by the game referee, the competition begins. The idea is to keep your stomach churning for as long as possible. Novices may be somewhat confused by the referees use of jargon and the use of such phrases as, "Churn away!" "Churn around!" and, at the end of the competition, "We've reached a Churning Point." However, hard-core bingers will seldom "churn down" the opportunity to play—even if they do not fully understand the rules of the game.

Things are too good

OBJECT OF THE GAME   To ruin things for yourself when things are going well.

HOW THE GAME IS PLAYED   If you've ever been thoroughly thrilled at getting a terrific new job, if you've ever experienced sweet infatuation or the genuine experience of love, if anything really great has ever happened to you—and if you have a problem binging—you've probably played this game. The game is played when the binger's own self-esteem keeps him or her from basking in accomplishment. The binger doesn't really believe that he or she deserves what has happened or there may be overwhelming guilt or anxiety associated with the good news.

Whatever, the answer to any and all problems associated with the good news is the same answer for problems that arise from other news—binge!

Through another's eyes

OBJECT OF THE GAME   To see yourself through another's eyes for the purpose of torturing yourself and prompting a binge.

HOW THE GAME IS PLAYED   If you are presently overweight, you may walk into a room and begin thinking that everyone is looking at your fat. If you are not overweight, you will walk in and think that everyone is noticing your inadequate hair, skin, or some other feature with which you are not comfortable. In any event, the result will be a binge. The key point to remember when playing this game is the importance of trying to infer what everyone is thinking about you and then futilely trying to live up to those standards. If you are to win at this game you must not set your own standards.

I know my rights!

OBJECT OF THE GAME   To assert your right to binge.

HOW THE GAME IS PLAYED   You may not have a legal right to commit suicide, but you certainly do have a legal right to binge. You can assert this right after you've been steadily dieting and taking off weight, after a major disappointment, even after a major victory. The point here is that you must shrug off the friendly concern of all those loved ones around you by asserting your constitutional right to binge. The player who gains the most weight as a result of asserting this right not only wins the game but can be authorized to hold an assertiveness-training workshop in his or her basement.

Just a taste

OBJECT OF THE GAME   To begin a binge by claiming to want only a taste of something that is not on your diet.

HOW THE GAME IS PLAYED   The play begins when someone around the binger is eating something the binger wants but should not really have.

"Can I have some of that?" the binger childishly asks.

"You know that you really shouldn't," comes the parentlike reply.

"How about just a taste?" the binger persists.

After the binger gets his or her way the binge begins. Because the binger now construes himself to be Off, all the stops are pulled and the binge officially begins.

Deprivation

OBJECT OF THE GAME   To deprive yourself of normal amounts of food and drink for five days or so and then make up for it all in approximately five minutes.

HOW THE GAME IS PLAYED   All competitors begin by swearing off most food forever. After about five days of quasi-fasting the players become moribund and decide that food isn't so bad after all. The "fast" is broken with a teaspoon of orange juice. Within the next two minutes or so the bingers' tolerance is such that spiced ham and provolone are no problem. By the end of three minutes the Deprived Bingers are already well into cheesecake and napoleons. At the end of five minutes all is back to "normal" and the game ends.

Hibernation

OBJECT OF THE GAME   To gain weight as a result of the lack of proper exercise.

HOW THE GAME IS PLAYED   Players of this game all know the value of proper exercise in any weight-control program. They are typically people who run, jog, swim, jump rope, or engage in some other form of exercise regularly. It is the change in seasons which signals the start of this game. At the beginning of the new season, players must think up reasons to postpone their exercise programs. Players might say they can't exercise because "it's too cold," "it's too hot," "it's too dark," or "it's too light." The player who gains the most weight as a result of cutting out all exercise is declared the winner. He or she wins a three-month supply of dried fruits and nuts.

Procrastination

OBJECT OF THE GAME   To binge when you have something important you must get done.

HOW THE GAME IS PLAYED   This is a game which can be played in your office or home. All that is required is that you have something very important to do (such as writing a report or a letter) which you really don't feel very much like doing. The play begins with the words "I'm hungry!" just when you are about to attack this task. The game ends when the task has been completed.

Bad taste

OBJECT OF THE GAME   To remedy the sensation of a bad taste by binging.

HOW THE GAME IS PLAYED   The play begins as soon as the bingers perceive a bad taste in the mouth. This game is frequently played when bingers first get up in the morning, when they get up in the middle of the night, when they are feeling ill, when they are taking medication, or after they have eaten a portion of Aunt Fanny's stuffed radishes. The winner is the player who gains the most weight trying to alleviate the bad taste with food. Prizes typically include a gallon of mouthwash, a six-pack of gum, and a package of breath/candy mints.

Love thy parents

OBJECT OF THE GAME   To show your parents how much you love them by binging.

HOW THE GAME IS PLAYED   This game begins when you go home to visit your parents. The rules say that all reason, common sense, and control must be left at the door. Your parents believe you have been starving while you haven't been living with them, and you cannot hurt their feelings by denying it. If your parents offer you something, you eat it to show them how much you love them. If there is a filled candy dish near where you happen to sit in the living room, you do not offend your parents by refusing the candy. If you are an overnight guest (or if you live with your parents), you can make up for any refusals to eat during the day by getting up and gorging yourself in the middle of the night. The winner is the player who gains the most weight after a specified length of time visiting their parents' home. First prize is a trophy with the inscription, "Good Son" or "Good Daughter" (whichever is appropriate). All players get consolation "care packages" to take home.

Great expectations

OBJECT OF THE GAME   To become discouraged and binge as a result of failing to live up to some great expectations.

HOW THE GAME IS PLAYED   Successful competitors in this game are those players who have set unrealistically high standards for themselves. They are seldom pleased with their accomplishments and believe that other people are too easily pleased with what they do. Almost any circumstance can prompt the initiation of this game. Great Expectations is frequently played shortly after bingers enroll in some weight-loss program. Players religiously attend meetings and carefully follow the program's prescribed diet for about three to five weeks. Soon players become discouraged that they are not losing weight as quickly as they (unrealistically) expect they should. This discouragement fosters the development of irrational thoughts like, "Dieting will never help *me*." Discouraged players then drive to the nearest French bakery where they immediately begin a new game, Eating for Two (see below).

Eating for two

OBJECT OF THE GAME   To trick the bakery clerk into believing you are shopping for more than one person.

HOW THE GAME IS PLAYED   The play begins when you get a yen for an eclair or a napoleon. You want to go into the bakery and buy one, but you really don't want the clerk to know it's for you. So instead of buying one, you buy a half dozen. This game is typically played in French bakeries (that is why it is sometimes referred to as The French Confection). Players may earn extra points if they drive up to the bakery, in full view of the clerk, in a station wagon. The winner is the player who has gained the most weight by "eating for two" (or more).

Nibbling

OBJECT OF THE GAME   To binge on empty-calorie foods when you aren't even hungry.

HOW THE GAME IS PLAYED   The play begins early in the evening as bingers comfortably position themselves in front of the television, making certain that an ample supply of empty-calorie snacks are within arm's length.* The idea is to consume large quantities of empty-calorie foods (usually in the form of sugars or animal fats) while not even thinking about what you are doing. A referee is needed for this binge game as the winner is the player who has accumulated the highest number of bites in a specified period of time. Players are cautioned against using foods that have textures similar to bananas when playing this game; it makes the scoring difficult.

London bridge

OBJECT OF THE GAME   To consume large quantities of food while thinking, "I can only get it here."

---

* Other versions of this game can be played on coffee breaks (in front of vending machines), at cookouts, even dinner parties. The only rule here is that all eating must be of a nonessential, "recreational" nature.

HOW THE GAME IS PLAYED   This game was created by a patient of mine who frequently commuted to London on business. There was this little bakery near a London bridge where they made a butter cookie that this man could not resist. He would eat mounds of them while in London thinking, "I can only get these cookies here." However, when he was ready to leave London, he would always be sure to bring home a two-month supply of these cookies for his freezer. Back in the States he would bring cookies as gifts to friends' houses and then wind up eating the majority of the gift himself.

People the world over play similar versions of London Bridge and, of course, you don't ever have to visit London to play. You can play London Bridge in Brooklyn, Scarsdale, even Bayonne, New Jersey. All you need to play is some special food from some special shop and a compelling, driving thought that goes something like, "I can only get it here, therefore I must gorge myself on it." For most people, tasting exotic foods that cannot usually be obtained close to home is a fun thing to do. However, for players of London Bridge, such tasting is not one of life's pleasures as much as it is a preoccupation and an obsession.

Penitence

OBJECT OF THE GAME   To repeat the phrase "I'll be better tomorrow" the most number of times before going on a binge.

HOW THE GAME IS PLAYED   All you will need to play this game is a box of your favorite cookies (*any* binge food will do) and the best of intentions for the following day. The game is played by saying the words "I'll be better tomorrow" in between every bite of every cookie.

Many Penitent Bingers find that playing Penitence on one day leads to playing it the next day too. The way it works is as follows: When a player gorges himself on Sunday he promises that he will be "good"* on Monday. Starving himself on Monday, he will be absolutely ravenous by Monday night. The Monday-night hunger will be accompanied by the thought, "Well, I was good all day today, therefore I am entitled to something to eat tonight." Eating to the point of fullness and beyond, moving slowly, breathing heavily, and just about ready to burst, players crawl into bed repeating the phrase "I'll be better tomorrow."

Free for all

OBJECT OF THE GAME   To eat as much as possible when there is an abundance of freely available food.

HOW THE GAME IS PLAYED   This is a game for bingers who tend to get carried away at weddings, wakes, Bar Mitzvahs— anyplace where there are copious quantities of food that is there for the binging. This game can also be played in all-you-can-eat restaurants, hotels with liberal second-serving policies, and in any room where a smorgasboard can be set up. Seasoned players starve themselves for hours before the competition so that they will not reach the point of nausea too soon after the festivities begin. Players come from many foreign countries and speak a variety of languages. The only requirement in this regard is that the terms "moderation," "self-control," and "sensible eating" be totally foreign to them.

Black magic

OBJECT OF THE GAME   To make calories taken in disappear into thin air.

---

* I do not approve of the use of the words "good," "legal," and other value-laden terms in weight-control programs. I prefer to simply ask my patients if they *deviated* from the program rather than asking if they were "good." Such value-laden terms can increase, exaggerate, and aggravate existing guilt feelings.

HOW THE GAME IS PLAYED No special wardrobe or props are required to play—capes and cauldrons are entirely optional. The trick here is to magically erase the calories from the foods you binge on so they will not be reflected on your scale. Some "magicians" believe they can make the calories disappear by only eating when standing. Others believe the calories will disappear into thin air if they binge along with a group and "everybody's doing it." Finally, there is a small group of magicians who believe that the calories will disappear so long as you smile broadly and elevate your shoulders with every bite of chocolate cake, ice cream, and related foods. Winners of Black Magic are the last to realize that when it comes to calories, they are incapable of performing a disappearing act. Despite their best efforts, the "thin air" will stay thin while they will not.

Spellbound

OBJECT OF THE GAME To experience a "spell" coming over you and to binge as a result.

HOW THE GAME IS PLAYED Players can be engaged in virtually any activity just before playing the game. They can, for example, be grooming their poodle, driving on the freeway, or blow drying their hair. The play begins when all of a sudden a "spell" comes over them and the urge to binge becomes strong. Some players have described the mysterious and mystical force that propels them into nonstop eating as an "ill wind" that came along (and their appetite control has gone with the wind). At such times many players feel "bewitched," and they rightly look to their family and friends for love and support in fighting off unwanted urges. In turning to others for help, the binger is acknowledging that breaking the "spell" is more a matter of exhortation than exorcism. Compassion and sensitivity from concerned people end this (and many other) binge games.

Dentist chair

OBJECT OF THE GAME To binge wildly on cold cuts before visiting the dentist.

HOW THE GAME IS PLAYED This game is played an hour or two before an appointment with your dentist. You know that you will be given a shot of novocaine and that you will not be able to eat for three or four hours afterwards. Anticipating your deprivation, you sit down with pre-dentist portions of ham, cheese, salami, and other cold cuts before leaving. Winners are the bingers who require the most dental work in one calendar year.

Red light, green light

OBJECT OF THE GAME To binge on red lights and to refrain from binging on green lights.

HOW THE GAME IS PLAYED This is a game played while driving in city streets. All you need is some high-calorie binge food next to you to keep you company. On red lights you can eat and on green lights you can't; it's as simple as that. The winner of this game is the player who gets the most red lights.

Cannibals

OBJECT OF THE GAME To use food as your trusted companion and then to eat your companion.

HOW THE GAME IS PLAYED The play begins when the binger starts taking chocolate chip cookies or other sweets along in the car to work, on the train to visit relatives, or anywhere else. The sweets begin to serve the purpose of a "companion" of sorts. Inevitably, the companion gets eaten and the binger must now get another companion.

Hearts and flowers

OBJECT OF THE GAME   To win as much sympathy as possible from your family and friends.

HOW THE GAME IS PLAYED   This game is played by bingers who tend not to have any sympathy for themselves. Instead, they have a bottomless pit for sympathy from others, and they will go around complaining how helpless they are in their eating habits in order to win that sympathy. Compulsive eaters want the world to sympathize with them. The winner of this game is the player who has manipulated the most people in his environment into expressing their condolences by sending sweet-smelling flowers and chocolate hearts.

Crumbs

OBJECT OF THE GAME   To be the first to pick up a crumb as soon as it hits the table.

HOW THE GAME IS PLAYED   A non-binger eating some crumbcake is seated at the head of a table with two binging players sitting on his right and left. The non-binger must eat the crumbcake in such a manner as to let all of the crumbs fall between the two players. Adequate perceptual-motor functioning is a must for the players who compete, for not only must they scoop up the falling crumbs but they must also consume them before scooping up anymore. The player to eat the most crumbs wins. It is parenthetically noted that those who play this game are typically content to play games in which they are satisfied with crumbs of emotional relationships as well.

Office in the kitchen

OBJECT OF THE GAME   To set up the kitchen as your primary place of business.

HOW THE GAME IS PLAYED   If at all possible, players who hold jobs in which they must leave their house should quit those jobs and take up some activity they can engage in exclusively in their kitchen. If it is not feasible to leave the job, the player must make it his business to spend as much time as humanly possible in the kitchen. This means reading in the kitchen, sewing in the kitchen, etc. Tempting foods should be kept conspicuously on display and snacks should be readily available. A player wins when he is spending the majority of his waking hours at home in the kitchen. First prize is a microwave oven.

Binge bingo

OBJECT OF THE GAME   To binge for five consecutive days on foods that start with the letter *B* on the first day, *I* on the second day, and so on.

HOW THE GAME IS PLAYED   The game begins when the players select five problem foods that begin with the letters *B*, *I*, *N*, *G*, and *O*. The next five days are spent binging wildly on these foods, each in their proper turn. The idea of this game is not to have any "free space" in your stomach.

Rationalization

OBJECT OF THE GAME   To think up the highest number of rationalizations or excuses for a binge.

HOW THE GAME IS PLAYED   The sample of rationalizations below is derived from some of the preceding material in this book. Try to enlarge the list by adding your favorites.

"I should binge because":

· I'm alone.
· I'm angry.
· I'm bored.
· I'm worried.
· It's a holiday.
· I'm not part of the group.
· I didn't have that much to eat today.
· I'm off.
· I'm going on a diet and must clean out the pantry.
· I'm beginning to look good.
· I'm feeling a little weak.
· I worked so hard preparing the meal.
· I want people to appreciate me for my brain.
· *Everybody's* doing it.
· I'm standing in the kitchen.
· I had a terrible time in traffic.
· I'm feeling self-destructive.
· I need to see a dentist.
· I'm beginning to look too good.

Charades

OBJECT OF THE GAME   To go through the motions of dieting while simultaneously binging.

HOW THE GAME IS PLAYED   Bingers who play charades must have their refrigerators well-stocked with mass quantities of diet ice cream, diet cake, diet soda, frozen yogurt, and the like. They may not use sugar in their coffee or other beverages though they may use sugar substitutes—even if they are having chocolate fudge cake with coffee! Charades is a long-term game in which the player is to act out the part of being on a diet while not making a serious commitment to weight loss through proper nutrition and exercise. This game is over when the binger realizes he has been playing games.

Miracle on Thirty-third Street

OBJECT OF THE GAME   To delegate responsibility for losing weight to some miracle method.

HOW THE GAME IS PLAYED   This game is usually played by huge masses of people. The game begins when all of the players assemble in Washington Square Park in New York City. Standing perfectly still, each of the players then tries to "meditate their fat away." Presumably, the fat is physically transported uptown to Thirty-third Street or thereabouts where it then dissipates.

If this game sounds totally silly to you remember this: It is no less silly than some of the miracle games you have played in the past. Fad "miracle" diets and exercise gimmicks are not solutions to the problem of *permanent* weight loss. Binging is a state of mind, not hunger. The only realistic solution is Awareness, Action, and Attitude.

Breaking the binge:

4

Awareness training

The first component in the AAA binge-breaking program is Awareness training. In the past, writers of self-help books have treated awareness the same way money has been treated. That is, everyone acknowledges you need it, but no one seems to have devised a very effective way of getting it. Dieters have been bombarded in print and on the air waves with words to the effect of "You have to gain an awareness." Further, the personnel at the local weight-reduction club, family physicians, and other community members can be relied upon to chide bingers for "not having an awareness" of what they are doing.

Talk is cheap. While there is no shortage of people telling you that you need to achieve an awareness of what you are doing, *there is a great shortage of people telling you how to achieve that awareness.* Psychologists and psychiatrists who specialize in the treatment of weight reduction are in the vast minority of mental health professionals. The self-proclaimed, untrained, and unlicensed weight "therapists" who can be found in any neighborhood are ill-equipped to provide effective tools. The grim fact is that the resources for achieving self-awareness are not available to the vast majority of weight-conscious people who are seeking specific and effective Awareness training.

What follows are some Awareness games—or perhaps more accurately some Awareness strategies—which you can begin to play if you are serious about losing weight. Use them to help pinpoint problem areas in your life and not as a substitute for personal psychological counseling.

Our Awareness training begins with two quizzes. The object of these two quizzes—and the rest of the Awareness and Action strategies to follow—is to help put you in touch with who you are and to help you to be all you can be.

Eating awareness quiz 1

Review Chapter 2 and answer the following questions:

1. How many of these binge types do I fall into? Which ones?
2. Can I see a future for myself where I no longer belong into any of these types?
3. How important is it to me to make binging one less problem in my life?

SCORING   Give yourself 100 points for each honest and correct answer. If you scored 300 you are already beginning to achieve some awareness and you are ready to continue.

Eating awareness quiz 2

Review Chapter 3 and answer the following questions:

1. How many of these binge games have I played? Which ones?
2. Can I see a future for myself where I am no longer playing binge games?
3. How important is it to me to never again play a binge game?

SCORING   Same as for quiz 1.

Calorie accountant

One of the most important strategies you can use to gain an awareness of your eating habits is to play Calorie Accountant. Just as financial accountants keep accurate records detailing money exchanges, a Calorie Accountant keeps accurate records detailing the quantity and caloric value of foods consumed. And just as accountants must be educated in the principles of accounting and the tools of their trade, so must a food accountant learn to weigh and measure food properly so estimates of caloric intake will be within a reasonable margin of error. Do not take it for granted that you know what a teaspoon of liquid is or what one ounce of "lean" meat looks like. Before playing Calorie Accountant, educate yourself with regard to all matters of weighing and measuring food. It is probably best to get this education in person—not from a book—so that you will be able to see the quantities you are talking about and have your questions answered. Contact the nutritionist at the hospital in your community to find out where you might be able to learn such weighing and measuring skills.

Once you have learned how to weigh and measure food you are ready to begin playing Calorie Accountant. The idea is to account for every morsel of food that passes your lips by writing down the quantity or amount of food eaten and the number of calories you have estimated that portion to contain. Keep accurate records by having a little notebook with you at all times. If you go out to eat make certain that every last morsel of food (right down to the last olive) gets recorded in your notebook. This doesn't mean you have to call attention to yourself by publicly writing everything down—you're not playing Public Accountant. What it means is that if you are serious this time about gaining an awareness—if you are going to do it this time —*everything* eaten at every hour of the day must be accounted for in your notebook. All of this information will be put to good use when you play Calorie Countdown, the action strategy described in Chapter 5.

Feelings accountant

A binge is a state of mind . . . not a state of hunger. Learning to tune in on your state of mind when you eat "normally" and when you binge is crucially important to your binge-breaking program. After you have played Calorie Accountant for about two weeks and you have begun to gain an awareness of your eating habits, it is time to make that awareness even more sophisticated. Feelings Accountant is an Awareness strategy that is actually an extension of Calorie Accountant. That is, in addition to continuing to keep careful records of the quantity and caloric value of the foods you eat, you will begin to keep accurate records of your feelings, emotions, and mood each time you pop something in your mouth. If you are ever to make binging a part of your past, you must learn to discriminate, recognize, and deal appropriately with such feelings as anger, depression, fatigue, boredom, and so on.

The tool of the Feelings Accountant's trade is a chart like the one on the next page. It is to be filled in daily and to be reread nightly. The information gained by playing Feelings Accountant will all be put to good use when you play Discrimination, the Action strategy described in Chapter 5.

Note that this chart also requires that you list the places in which you consumed the food and the people who were around you at the time. All of this is designed to do just one thing: Provide you with a lifelong awareness of your eating habits. You may find you eat more high-calorie foods in the presence of your husband than you do at other times. You may find you eat the most food when you are at your parents' home or when you are visiting your grandmother in the hospital. Are you eating more when you feel "dizzy" than when you feel "okay"? There is a wealth of information to be obtained from the Daily Record Chart. Start your AAA binge-breaking program off on the right foot by taking the time and effort to keep your records accurate and current.

We have recommended that you spend about two weeks playing Calorie Accountant and an additional two weeks playing Feelings Accountant. In this regard one point cannot be overemphasized: *Do not diet or in any way modify your usual*

Daily record chart of the Feelings Accountant

TIME	PLACE	PEOPLE AROUND ME	FOOD EATEN	QUANTITY	CALORIES	FEELINGS

and *"normal" eating patterns for the month you will be account-ing for your food and feelings!** The purpose of playing ac-countant is to gain insight into what your eating habits have been. If you modify your eating habits in any way before playing accountant, the data you collect will be virtually useless. *It is imperative that you refrain from dieting for about a month if you are ever to gain an awareness of the meaning food has for you.* Many weight patients find this beginning stage of the binge-breaking program difficult to accept. They come to the program "raring to go," and they do not like to be told it will be a month before they will enter the second (action) stage of treatment. I instruct my patients that the month they spend gaining an awareness of themselves may pay off royally in pounds lost and kept off in the future. I usually say something like, "You have yo-yo'd back and forth so long, isn't it time you spent some time to reflect?"

The rest of the games in this chapter can be played (or modified to be played) either before or after your initial month of Awareness training.† Our goal in this binge-breaking program is to help you develop a binge-free lifestyle you can live with— *not just loss of weight!* To help yourself toward that goal, you must know where you are going. And before you know where you are going, you must know where you are at. Awareness training is the first step in finding where you are.

Demolition derby

The idea of this game is to demolish all myths about weight loss. Begin by demolishing the idea that weight control by *any*

---

* This is not a license to binge! It is simply an instruction to continue eating in the way you have been eating in the past.

† The one Awareness game which cannot be played simultaneously with Calorie or Feelings Accountant is Kiss My 200s Goodbye; it is an Aware-ness game that is played once you are well on your "weigh" to weight loss.

method can be "quick and easy." Next, demolish the idea that your excess weight or your binging ways have been brought on by defective glands, hormones, or genes. Although you should have a good physical exam to rule out such causes of binging, be aware of the fact that you are in the minority if your obesity is due to some real physical defect. For most bingers, the only problem is an overactive *salivary* gland brought about by conscious decisions to eat!

Another myth that must be demolished is the one that equates being thin with being sickly. One of my male patients who lost a great deal of weight had to put up with being greeted by his family and friends with lines like, "Gee, John, you lost a lot of weight, are you feeling all right?" It is true that a sudden, unexplainable loss in weight can be a sign of disease, but probably not when you are conscientiously trying to lose.

It's hard to believe, but some people still equate being heavy with being wealthy. Actually, it's probably the other way around. That is, wealthy people have more time to engage in sports and other recreational activities and usually have many more diversions to keep them occupied. Still, the idea that overweight people are wealthy persists. One patient of mine burst with pride as she described the fullness of her pantry and refrigerator. She said that she was proud of the fact that her married children could do their food shopping for the week at her house if they wanted to. A first step in helping this woman to obtain a healthy awareness of herself and what food represented to her was to help her demolish the myths she clung to concerning food, dieting, and losing weight.

Stop, look, and listen

Think back to all of the times you've stopped yourself from binging. Your immediate response might be, "I've never stopped myself from a binge." However, if you think hard enough you will be able to recall some time when you thought you were going to binge but you suddenly decided not to. Everyone has one private thought that is capable of stopping them from binging. The idea of this game is to Stop, Look, and Listen to your better judgment when you think you might indulge in a binge. Your better judgment is *your* better judgment and no one elses. Therefore no one can tell you what you should do to turn on the Stop mechanism. However, the Stop mechanism for some of my patients have been thoughts like:

· "I know I am going to be sick with diabetes."
· "I'm not going to be able to breathe."
· "I won't have anything to wear."
· "I'm going to feel more depressed afterwards so I will not do this to myself."

Everyone has a Stop mechanism—even the most "hard-core" bingers. What is yours?

Truth and consequences

The object here is to develop an awareness of the consequences of your actions.

· Ask yourself now, "What will be the consequences if I do not change my eating habits?"
· Ask yourself before beginning a binge, "What will be the consequences of this binge?"
· Ask yourself in a quiet moment of contemplation, "What will be the consequences of my weight loss?"

Truthfully answer each of these questions and write your answers on index cards. Have the index cards ready when you feel a binge coming on. If you have been honest with yourself it will be more difficult to binge in good conscience after you've re-read those cards.

What's wrong with this picture?

Countless weight patients that I've treated complain of some "unconscious block" that is stopping them from losing weight and living a binge-free existence. It is for those patients that I developed the What's-Wrong-With-This-Picture? game. I usually employ this technique when the patient is deeply hypnotized, but you probably don't have to be deeply hypnotized for it to work. All you do is lie back in a comfortable chair, allow yourself to completely relax, and visualize a scene in which you are at your goal weight. The scene should be so vividly visualized that you can see every detail of the clothing you are wearing and feel as good as you might when you reach your goal weight. Introduce your spouse and/or other friends and family into the scene and see yourself engaged in conversation with them.

As you get more deeply involved in this scene, you should experience a sense of uneasiness, a sense that something is not quite right. For example, one woman I treated perceived herself basically as a very "earthy" person. Only when we used the What's-Wrong-With-This-Picture? technique did she become aware of the fact that she equated being slim with being sophisticated and snobby. This greatly upset her because she was not able to see herself having any friends. The use of this technique thus served to break through a major block in this woman's lifelong battle of the binge.

We will have more to say about the What's-Wrong-With-This-Picture? technique when we talk about reaching a Moment of Truth in your life. Right now, try to visualize yourself thin and come up with an answer to the question, "What's wrong with this picture?"

Is the price right?

Your body is a very efficient organism that uses all of the energy that is put into it. It may use that energy to perform routine functions such as keeping your heart beating, keeping your lungs breathing, etc.,* or it may use that energy for activities like mowing the lawn, jogging, and any other function that occurs when the body is not in a state of rest. Food provides energy to the body. The energy that isn't used is efficiently stored in the form of fat. When the diet is out of balance and/or when the energy put out by the body is far less than the energy put in, more and more fat will accumulate. Scientists tell us that the more excess fat we carry around with us, the more likely we are to suffer from heart trouble, gall bladder trouble, kidney trouble, arthritis, and diabetes. Statistics indicate that a middle-aged man who weighs only twenty-five pounds above what he should weigh has decreased his life expectancy by twenty-five percent. Numerous other physical, psychological, and social problems that work to shorten the obese person's life expectancy are a daily reality.

If you are obese and if you engage in frequent binging, play Is the Price Right? during your next binge to help reinforce your awareness of the self-destructive nature of the act in which you are engaging. The game is played by asking yourself just before consuming every forkful, spoonful, or handful, "Is the price right?" Make this game as short as possible.

---

* The amount of energy your body uses to perform these basic functions is called the "basal metabolism rate." The rate differs from person to person and is dependent upon your body size, health, as well as other factors.

Test of strengths

This is a game for those bingers who for countless years have preferred to play games that give them an opportunity to expose their weaknesses. In Test of Strengths the binger has one whole evening to sit down and list his strong points. What are your strengths?

· Are you able to mix well with others and put them at ease when you meet them?
· Are you handy around the house?
· Is your greatest strength your determination to get a job done once you decide it's worth doing?
· Is your ability to achieve peace with yourself a strength of yours?
· Does your tolerance for other people number within your strengths?
· Is your knowledge within your chosen profession your greatest strength?

Becoming aware is very much a process of coming to know your strengths as well as your weaknesses.

Gourmet

This is a game played to heighten one's awareness of the taste, smell, and texture of food. The game is played over a course of one week. Everything that is taken into the mouth is put on the right side of the tongue then the left side of the tongue. All portions are cut in half then in half again before they go into the mouth. The idea here is to taste food to the fullest, to savor it, to love it, and *not have to binge on it*. Bingers typically swallow food for the sole purpose of making way for more. In Gourmet, bingers learn to truly taste and delight in food.

PERSONal touch

Awareness means not only being aware of yourself as simply a fat person, a thin person, or a person with problem eating habits; it means being aware of yourself as a *person*. A *person* has needs, hopes, dreams, fears, aspirations, imperfections, and requirements. There's a lot to you besides your weight, there's more to think about than simply your eating habits, and there's more to talk about than diets, food, weight, eating, and dress sizes. Fat or thin, rich or poor, young or old you are a *person* who must love, respect, and protect yourself. And if right now you do happen to have an overeating problem, make sure to convey to the people around you that you are treating yourself as a person and that there is a lot more to you than your dress size.

Fencing

This game is designed to provide you with an awareness of what you are doing everytime you go to the refrigerator or pantry. In order to play, you will have to buy some brightly colored ribbons and fence off a portion of your pantry and your refrigerator with it. A red ribbon would be most appropriate because red is associated with "Stop," and this is the message you will eventually want to get. Within the fenced areas you are to put all of the foods you are buying and storing within the house that you know you should not eat. Remember that the purpose of the fenced area is not to stop you from eating—even barbed wire couldn't do that—only to remind you and give you an awareness of what you are doing.

Kentucky doily

Another consciousness-raising game, Kentucky Doily is played on a placemat with a doily directly alongside. All of your eating at home, whether it is on your diet, off your diet, on a binge, or whatever must be done on the same placemat with the doily. The presence of the placemat and the doily will serve to "anchor" all of your eating and make you all the more conscious of what you are doing. Make sure not to watch television, read, listen to the radio, or engage in any other competing activity while playing this game. The only thing that can be done simultaneously with the eating is some social conversation.

Gag

This is an Awareness strategy for bingers who play games while they are preparing food. The idea here is to wear a gag while cooking. Note that the gag is not designed to stop the binger from eating. The binger may in fact remove the gag if he so desires to sample foods while engaged in food preparation or even to binge for that matter. The wearing of the gag during food preparation periods is done for the sole purpose of allowing the binger to be free from "unconscious" binging. The rules of the game provide that the gag can only be removed for one taste at a time. This game is of course not for bingers whose physical health would be impaired by the wearing of the gag. It is for bingers whose health may be more impaired if they do not wear it.

Bridge

This is an exciting game that allows the player to add a lot of leather to his wardrobe if he plays his cards right. Everytime the binger "crosses the bridge" from one size to a lower size, a "Bridge" is declared and the binger is allowed to reward himself with a new leather belt in the new size. The game continues until the player reaches his goal size. Water weight gains during the course of this game do not compel a player to forfeit any prizes. Rather, such weight gains are appropriately looked upon as simply "water under the bridge."

New math

Contrary to what you might expect, New Math is not a game of numbers. Rather it is an Awareness game, the object of which is to determine what adds up to what for you. For example, you may find that *Anger* plus *Frustration* equals *Calories*. Or you might be surprised to learn that *Contentment with Self* minus *Spouse's Attention* equals *Binge*. What's your "binge quotient"? Take some time with this game and do some "figuring" in order to determine what factors in your life add up to problem eating habits. When you think you've calculated the right answer, count on no one but yourself to correct the equation. If you play New Math seriously, your binge days will be numbered.

7 minutes in heaven

The idea of this Awareness game is to get excited, hot, and bothered at the thought of yourself thin. Set your alarm clock to go off about seven minutes from the time you begin this game. Then begin to fantasize how "heavenly" you will look without all the unwanted pounds. And don't just think of yourself thin or picture yourself a few sizes down, make sure to *get yourself excited* at the prospect of being that thin. Allow seven minutes of each day until you reach your goal weight to put yourself "in heaven." Most importantly, build into your weight-loss program sufficient rewards and future plans to ensure that when you reach your goal weight the once nightmarish hell of being overweight doesn't again begin to look more attractive.

Kiss my 200s goodbye

This game is a kind of farewell party designed to ceremoniously say good riddance to a part of you that was part of your past. The game is played everytime you lose at least ten pounds and cross the line from one weight that is a denomination of ten to another. For example, you would play Kiss My 200s Goodbye when you crossed the line from 200 to 199. You would play Kiss My 190s Goodbye when you crossed the line from 190 to 189, and so forth. A frequently worn article of old clothing is "It," and "It" is passed around to each of the players who are seated in a circle in your living room. The clothing article represents your old weight, and each of the players must kiss "It" goodbye (passionate kissing is discouraged) and give a brief spiel designed to welcome the "new" you. All of this should help you to acquire a greater awareness and acceptance of yourself at your new weight and help you to lay your old weight to rest with dignity. Screening of players for mononucleosis is entirely optional.

Contagious outlooks

What do you know that spreads more easily than good feelings and a positive attitude? Jennifer, one of my former patients, learned the value of an optimistic attitude in helping not only herself in her weight-loss program but also her husband. When she was well into therapy Jennifer came in one day and said, "Since my attitude toward food has changed my husband has lost fifteen pounds." Contagious Outlooks is a game that can only be played by persons who are ready and capable to sacrifice pessimism for optimism and depression for conviction. Are you ready to play?

Stitch-in-time

This is a time-consuming game but one that should pay off in a weight loss and a binge-free attitude that is *maintained*. The idea is to develop an awareness and acceptance of the fact that permanent weight loss and an unshakable binge-free attitude can only be acquired over time. Exactly how long it will take to develop in each individual person is unique to that person's life history and present-life circumstances. However, you can be sure that it will not be developed in one day, one week, or one month. To play Stitch-in-Time, circle dates on your calendar by which you wish to achieve certain goal weights and certain attitudes. *Allow yourself time to lose the weight*, never estimating more than one and a half to two and a half pounds per week. Similarly, be liberal with yourself in terms of your planned attitude changes. For example, do not resolve something like, "By the first of next month I will hate ice cream." Say instead, "By the first of next month I will love ice cream as much as I always have, but I will love myself a little more and therefore be able to cut my intake of ice cream substantially." Common sense and the ability to plan realistic goals are all that are necessary to play Stitch-in-Time.

Excess baggage

Almost everyone is carrying some kind of excess baggage in terms of some self-defeating mental attitude or way of behaving. Such excess baggage can "weigh you down" not only in terms of a weight-loss program but in life in general. The idea of Excess Baggage is to gather up all of your own unneccessary baggage and leave it behind. What's your excess baggage? Is it guilt? Is it anger? Let close friends and family help you in becoming aware of what it is and how you might go about leaving it behind. In severe cases, you may want to see a psychologist or other mental health professional for assistance in becoming aware of (and eventually dealing with) your excess baggage.

Bayonne, New Jersey

This is a game to help you become aware of how good things are in your life. The game is played whenever you think things are really bad, whenever you are really down, and whenever you believe you knocked on Fate's door and nobody was home. Whenever things seem to be at their absolute worst, that is the time to do one thing: Just think how much worse your lot would be if you lived in Bayonne, New Jersey. This is a strategy that was suggested to me by a patient who used to have anxiety attacks every time she drove through the Holland Tunnel. Everyone has a city they can't stand. For W.C. Fields it was Philadelphia. Whether he was in New York, Hollywood, Chicago, or anywhere else, Fields could be heard to say, "Better here than in Philadelphia." In fact, engraved on the tombstone of W.C. Fields are the words, "Better here than in Philadelphia."

Reward or consolation?

Think about the last time you went shopping and bought yourself a few things. Now ask yourself: Did I buy those things to reward myself or to console myself? If you say "neither," give it a little bit more thought and ask yourself what you generally do. If you have come to the conclusion that you went shopping to reward yourself, this is a good sign of your ability to be goal-oriented and to pay yourself off for achieving those goals. If you are shopping to console yourself, you may not be dealing constructively with the problems for which you are consoling yourself. In any case, part of losing weight and developing an anti-binge orientation is rewarding yourself (with nonfood rewards) for getting things done. Self-consolation does have a place in life, but it is no substitute for achievement of realistic goals and effective problem solving. Gain an awareness of your shopping habits by asking yourself from time to time, "Did I buy this to reward or to console myself?"

What's important to me?

There are many ways to embark on a weight-loss program. One is to approach it by saying, "This is just another program." Another way is to say, maybe somewhat half-heartedly, "I'll give it a try." Perhaps the most constructive way to begin any program designed to culminate in weight loss and an anti-binge orientation is to ask yourself, "What's important to me?" Is weight loss and a binge-free life *really* important to you? Or is the feeling of mounds of chocolate cake and ice cream lining your mouth and throat more important? You must make a decision, if not for your own welfare then for the welfare of your children, spouse, friends, and the others around you.

I am loved
I am prized
I am needed
I have the self-esteem to stick
with this!

In the beginning you can make a game of saying these four reminders to yourself every morning. Once they become permanently etched onto your brain the game is over. You will be free from the need to engage in self-destructive acts.

Breaking the binge:

Action strategies

Action is the second component of the AAA method of binge-breaking. To understand what is meant by Action, let us state clearly what it is *not:* Action is not "tomorrow."

Anything worth taking action on is worth taking action on today. If it is medically safe for you to begin to lose weight, anti-binge Action must begin *now,* even as you read these words. Now is not after the weekend, after vacation, after Aunt Lilly's affair, or after anything else . . . "now" means *now.*

ACTION IS NOT JUST A DIET

You've probably had your fill of diets and diet programs in which the only person who benefited was the person or group offering the diet. Any program that offers you a diet without personalized psychological help is doomed to achieving from partial to no success at all. This is so because, as we will point out again and again, a binge is a state of mind, not a state of hunger.

ACTION IS NOT A FAD APPROACH TO WEIGHT LOSS

At one time you may have believed that if you just sent away for some gimmick diet or exercise device you would lose weight and keep it off. But experience has probably taught you there is no pill, liquid, powder, girdle or belt, exercise apparatus, or medical procedure that will miraculously transform you into a slim person. Of course you will probably lose weight on even the most ridiculous of these fad approaches, but you will just as certainly gain it right back after varying lengths of time. Fad approaches seldom if ever encourage balanced nutrition and exercise and never deal with faulty attitudes and behaviors.

Moreover, most fad diets cannot be followed for extended periods of time because they are either impractical or downright boring.

In all too many cases, fad diets arouse intensely negative feeling states that sooner or later culminate in extended binging which ultimately wipes out any progress made in weight reduction. The rage of the person who has had his jaws wired together for an extended period of time will at one time or another express itself in a binge once the jaws are unwired. The person who must drink some awful tasting potion instead of enjoying a finely prepared meal with friends, family, or coworkers is likely to feel deprived, left out, or even punished. All of these fad approaches to the complex problem of weight loss have the paradoxical effect of making food all the more attractive to the fad dieter.

ACTION IS NOT AN INCOMPLETE APPROACH TO WEIGHT LOSS

Awareness, proper nutrition, proper exercise, proper attitude, and the proper structuring of your environment are all part of what is meant by constructive Action. Incomplete approaches to weight loss are approaches that overemphasize one or another of these parts to the de-emphasis or exclusion of another. For example, some hypnotists will focus exclusively on the awareness component and not give proper attention to the other components. Hypnosis, it should be said, does have a place in a weight-control program for those persons who want it and can profit from it. However, its place is that of an adjunct to treatment, *not* as a treatment in itself. Persons or programs who rely exclusively on hypnosis as a method of treatment, especially impersonal hypnosis (hypnosis by tapes or records), are building failure into their treatment and wasting your time and money.

ACTION: WHAT IS IT?

Action means resolving today to make the battle of the binge one less battle in your life. Action means trading in binge games for Awareness strategies and the sacrifice of poor eating/exercise habits. Strategies for effective Action follow. Although we will treat these strategies as "games," so that they will be fun to carry out, do not lose sight of the fact that Action is very serious business!

Calorie countdown

It takes 3500 extra calories to make your bathroom scale register one more pound of weight on you. Over the course of a week that's 3500 divided by seven or only 500 extra calories per day. This means that if your caloric needs were, for example, 2000 calories per day and you were taking in 2500 calories per day, you would be gaining one pound of weight per week (all things such as exercise output being equal).

But just as it takes 3500 calories more than you need to put on an extra pound, it also takes 3500 calories less per week for you to lose one pound a week. So here is the good news: If you take in just 500 calories less per day than you need, you will be losing a pound of weight per week. If you take in 750 calories less per day you will be losing one and a half pounds per week, 1000 calories less, two pounds, and so on.

Suppose after you've played the awareness game Calorie Accountant you realized that you were averaging a caloric intake of 2750 calories per day. That's quite a lot of calories! To go from an average of 2750 calories per day to an average of 1200 per day, as some weight programs expect you to do, would probably be too great a step for you to take all at once and failure would automatically be built into your weight program. However, if you could modify your caloric intake by taking in just 750 calories less per day (that would be an intake of 2000 calories per day in this case) you should lose one and a half pounds per week. And 2000 calories per day is quite a large number of calories to play with! All you need to play Calorie Countdown is your data from Calorie Accountant and the food-weighing and measuring skills you have acquired and become proficient at.

Student-exchange program

After successfully playing Calorie Countdown for about two weeks or so you will be ready to move on to a program of exchange dieting. To do so, you will have to become a student of food-exchange groups. Your teacher will be the nutritionist you contacted when you were learning the weighing and measuring skills needed to play Calorie Accountant. If you have never had a consultation with a nutritionist and you are serious about making your lifestyle consistent with your bodily needs, an appointment with one is an excellent idea. The time and money you spend for the consultation will be well worth the gains in personal awareness and the good health which comes from intelligent eating habits. Supplementing the nutritional advice, a booklet on Exchange-List Dieting that is published jointly by the American Dietetic Association and the American Diabetes Association may be useful to you.* The six lists contained in the booklet include milk exchanges, vegetable exchanges, fruit exchanges, bread exchanges, meat exchanges, and fat exchanges.

Exchange-list dieting takes the boredom out of watching your weight because it allows you to substitute a variety of foods within each of the food groupings for a number of other foods. The beauty of it all is that you can have practically anything

---

* The booklets are made available for less than $1 each. Contact the American Diabetes Association, Inc., 1 West 48th Street, New York, N.Y. 10020 or the American Dietetic Association, 430 North Michigan Avenue, Chicago, Illinois 60611 for more information.

you want—in moderation of course. No longer must you feel guilty about putting mayonnaise on your sandwich—go right ahead and write it off as a fat exchange. The important psychological advantage to exchange dieting is that you no longer feel deprived and you no longer feel guilty. There is a whole universe of delectable "diet food" beyond lettuce, tuna fish, and cottage cheese, and you should discover it! If you have special dietary needs (e.g., low-sodium diet, sugar-restricted diet, etc.), it would be a good idea to check with your doctor and design an exchange list that will be right for you. It is always a good idea to check with your doctor anyway before embarking on this or any other weight-control program.

Let's make some deals

This Action strategy is designed to help you play Calorie Countdown and Student-Exchange Program. The rules are simple: Make up a "Reward List" and give yourself a reward for every week your average caloric intake has been within the limit you set for yourself in Calorie Countdown. Your Reward List may contain material things (such as a bottle of expensive perfume), activities (a long-distance phone call to your sister in Hawaii; fifteen minutes of massage from your spouse)—*anything* that you find rewarding. Of course, the fact that you are sticking to your AAA program will be rewarding in its own right. Still, these extra little rewards along the way can help to keep motivation high, especially in the beginning stages.

Let's Make Some Deals should be played for the first two months of the Action stage of the AAA program. After two months you will move on to playing Once Can Be Enough (see below). One word of caution: When playing Let's Make Some Deals, *do not make rewards contingent on weight loss!* This is a major mistake that many weight-program leaders and therapists make early in weight-control programs. Patients and clients begin weight-control programs with high hopes of losing weight quickly and when they do not, they become discouraged. Therefore, Let's Make Some Deals makes the rewards contingent on your report of caloric intake, *not* on weight loss. Weight fluctuates at various times during the month, and this fluctuation may have no reliable correlation with food intake. Making rewards contingent on weight loss in the beginning of treatment may be building into the program unnecessary feelings of frustration. I have found that after approximately two months of Let's Make Some Deals, patients can then safely begin rewarding themselves for weight loss.

Once can be enough

Like Let's Make Some Deals, Once Can Be Enough is an Action strategy designed to help you along in your AAA binge-breaking program. In this game you are to weigh yourself once a week on the same scale at the same time, preferably with no clothes on. The key word here is *once*. Some people weigh themselves seven or more times a week to see if their dieting has registered on their bathroom scale. These people set themselves up for disappointment because reduced food intake does not automatically register as pounds lost. Once Can Be Enough means never having to be disappointed (well, almost never). Remember: "once" does not mean weighing yourself after jogging for an hour, fasting (or feasting) for a day, or right after making love with "Fast" Irwin from the Bronx. "Once" means *once* a week.

After you have begun to play this game, you can begin to reward yourself for weight loss. Exactly how many pounds you must lose to obtain a reward is entirely up to you. However, it makes sense to "up" the value of the rewards as you go down in weight. It is a good idea to graph your weekly progress. Pages 102–105 is a sample "Once Can Be Enough" chart. Notice that various rewards have been marked in for achieving certain weights.* Also notice that when the goal weight is reached, rewards are given for maintaining that weight.

Discrimination

In playing the Awareness game Feelings Accountant, you learned to tune in on your state of mind when you ate "normally" and when you binged. In the Action strategy Discrimination, it is time to put the information to good use. Take out your Daily Record Chart of the Feelings Accountant which you kept for a two-week period. What patterns can you discern? When are your problem eating times? in whose company? Do you eat more or less when you are alone? Do you eat more or less when you are home or away from home? What kinds of food do you eat when you are with people, away from home, and it is late at night? What kinds of feelings do you experience when you are alone at home? alone away from home? Is there a difference in your state of mind during problem and nonproblem eating periods?

Playing Discrimination means more than being aware of the relationship between problem eating habits and feelings; it means *acting* to remedy the problem. Once you have learned to discriminate boredom from fatigue and anger from depression, for example, you must work on responding appropriately to these feelings. If you experience a feeling of hunger you will eat. However, if you are bored, you will deal with the boredom and not eat. Remedies for boredom are a matter of personal

---

* The rules of the game say that you cannot be rewarded for achieving the same weight twice. That is, if you give yourself a pedicure for reaching a weight of 200, you can't give yourself another pedicure for gaining and then returning to 200.

"Once Can Be Enough" weight-loss and reward chart

WEIGHT	WEEK OF [Pencil dates in brackets below]	REWARD

[ ] [ ] [ ] [ ] [ ] [ ] [ ] [ ] [ ]

210
209
208 ●
207 ●
206 ●
205 ●
204 ●
203 ● Beauty parlor (no facial)
202
201
200
199
198
197 Pedicure
196
195
194
193

Beauty parlor and facial

15 minutes of conversation with husband

15 minutes of conversation with someone else (such as a close friend or relative)

192
191
190
189

188
187
186
185
184
183

182
181
180
179
178
177

176
175
174
173
172
171

"Once Can Be Enough" weight-loss and reward chart [Continued]

WEIGHT	WEEK OF [Pencil dates in brackets below] [ ] [ ] [ ] [ ] [ ] [ ] [ ] [ ]	REWARD
170		
169		Backrub from husband
168		
167		
166		
165		
164		
163		
162		
161		Backrub from someone else
160		
159		
158		
157		Buy expensive handbag
156		
155		
154		

153
152
151
150

Night at swank nightclub with husband (or someone else)

MAINTENANCE

1 week   Beauty parlor (full treatment)

1 month   New shoes

2 months   New underwear

3 months   New wardrobe

6 months   Trip to visit sister in Hawaii

preference but you might try watching television, crocheting, reading a good book, taking a walk, writing a poem, or calling a friend. If you are fatigued you will not eat but lie down, take a nap, meditate, etc. Once you have become a Certified Feelings Accountant, you will have the knowledge and skill to discriminate your feelings. It is comforting to know that with a little practice in acting appropriately on those feelings, a binge-free future can be in the offing.

Anticipation

A binge-breaking strategy that my patients have found most appealing, Anticipation involves writing down everything you eat with the caloric value of the food . . . *before* you eat it. Buy a large notebook. In the beginning, write everything down a few minutes before you actually sit down to eat. Make sure to include the quantity of the food and an accurate estimate of the calories you are about to take in. With time, you should be able to plan your day's menu the night before. Whether you need to plan your menus more than a day in advance is something you will have to decide for yourself after personal experimentation. The important thing is to write everything down in your notebook *before* you eat it. Even if you spontaneously and impulsively decide to deviate from your planned menu (it happens and it's not the end of the world!), make certain to write down what you are going to eat before you eat it.

One of my patients not only writes down everything in her Anticipation notebook, she also writes it down on a slip of paper. The paper is then placed under a plastic, translucent placemat on which she eats all her meals at home. While eating, she takes pleasure from knowing she is keeping to the structure she has set for herself. Whether a translucent placemat should be a permanent fixture in your home is, again, a matter of personal preference. What is important is that you write down everything before you eat it . . . *everything*.

Competing activities

Competing activities are so called because the activity they compete with is binging. "How do I play Competing Activities?" you ask. The answer is *get involved* in something that interests you, something other than food. Some Competing Activities you might try include knitting; embroidery; gardening; driving; listening to music; taking up a musical instrument; donating time to a local hospital, charity, or political campaign; writing; jumping rope; going swimming; getting involved in political functions; calling businesses in the phone directory and asking about their goods and services; cleaning out your drawers or closets; dropping your faraway friends a line; taking a course; taking a bike ride; reading; drawing; walking; taking up ceramics; taking up acting, dancing, or singing; going to the ballet; teaching your old dog some new tricks . . . the list is virtually endless. One of my patients bought a loom and began making potholders (instead of holding pots). One hundred potholders later, she had raised a tidy sum for her charitable organization and lost twenty-three pounds in the bargain.

PERSONal growth

In the Awareness game, *Person*al Touch, we suggested that you get in touch with other aspects of your life besides your problem eating habits and/or your weight. Here we suggest that your newfound personal awareness can be complemented by *Person*al Growth. *Person*al Growth is a logical extension of the anti-binge

Action strategy, Competing Activities. When a competing activity ceases to be a competing activity, you have *Personal* Growth. For example, suppose you take up knitting as an activity to compete with binging; every time you feel like binging you would pick up your knitting. But at some point you may find yourself picking up your knitting even when you don't feel like binging. In fact, you may find you get tremendous satisfaction and a feeling of accomplishment from your knitting. Almost any activity—from dropping your friend a line to cleaning out your drawers—has potential for *Personal* Growth.

18½-minute gap

This Action game should be most beneficial to you in both the initial and later stages of binge-breaking. The game involves taking an 18½-minute pause, when the urge to binge comes over you, to do anything you wish instead of eating. The best way to play 18½-Minute Gap is to have a list of activities in which you can engage when the urge comes. A good thing about playing this game is that right after you're through playing it once, there's no harm in playing it again. Many people report that it is getting by just the first few minutes of a "binge feeling" that is important; if they can get past those first few minutes by engaging in a non-binge or anti-binge activity, they've got that binge licked!

Glutton for punishment

The qualities necessary to successfully play Glutton for Punishment are good mental imagery, a strong desire to control impulsivity, and an educated ability to become nauseous on command. The key to winning this Action strategy is a capacity to mentally *exaggerate* the consequences of participating in any of the binge games in Chapter 3. For example, suppose you have been playing Commercial Vehicle for more days than you care to remember. The next time a tempting commercial comes on television and you are about to be propelled into the kitchen, stop and play Glutton for Punishment: Stop and imagine yourself eating not one or two of the product being advertised but ten or twenty of them. Close your eyes and *feel* as if you have just eaten ten or twenty of them. You should begin to experience the actual nausea that you would really feel if you had eaten that much. Open your eyes when the commercial goes off and let the nausea quickly dissipate. You should feel better for not having punished yourself with snacks and for having gained a sense of mastery over a previously threatening situation. The principle on which this strategy is based can be applied to most any problem. All it takes is a little imagination—and exaggeration.

Slowly but surely

Like the preceding Action strategy, the object of this game is to put yourself in control of situations that you may not have had control of in the past. However, whereas the principle involved in Glutton for Punishment is exaggeration, the primary principle in Slowly But Surely is *gradual exposure* to situations that have triggered past binges. Again using the binge game Commercial Vehicle as an example, let us see how Slowly But Surely could be effectively used as an anti-binge strategy.

Players are instructed to watch television for shorter periods of time than usual and only when their stomachs are full. The latter part of this rule assures that players will not be exposing themselves to problem situations when they might think they are hungry. If a player felt any given commercial was threatening his control, he could quickly change channels to the educational television station in his area (simply because there are no commercials there). After watching educational television for a minute or so the player could turn back to what he was originally watching. In the beginning, television watching should be restricted to about one hour as close to after-dinner time as possible. Add half an hour of television watching every two weeks. After only a few short months you should be able to watch any commercial on television, even when you are hungry, without having to run into the kitchen and without having to turn on educational television. *By gradually increasing your exposure to a previously threatening situation you have gained a sense of control and mastery.*

As another example, suppose you have been a regular player of If I'm in the Kitchen I Must Be Hungry. Again, Slowly But Surely may be the anti-binge Action strategy of choice for you. To play, you begin by "psyching yourself up" for trips into the kitchen in which you would do nothing but stand there for about a minute or two. Make sure that such initial trips are during "safe" time periods, such as right after dinner, when you are not at all hungry and when you are well aware of why you are going into the kitchen. Experience how good it feels to be in control of a situation in which you lacked such control in the past. Increase your exposure time daily by about half a minute or so until you can spend about seven minutes in the kitchen without touching the refrigerator or pantry. The next month repeat the process, beginning this time half an hour after dinner, the following month one hour after dinner, and so on. If you get stuck along the way, go back to the point you were at two weeks before.

It will take patience and dedication for this anti-binge Action strategy to be effective against Commercial Vehicle, If I'm in the Kitchen I Must Be Hungry, or any other binge game.

However, the joy of control can be yours if you are willing to play Slowly But Surely.

Figure skating

Improving your figure by skating or any other form of regular exercise can be fun as well as healthful. However, as with dieting, you should check with your physician before beginning any exercise regimen. Once you've gotten a clean bill of health, there's an exciting world of sports and competition awaiting you. Besides Figure Skating there are numerous other exercise-related games. You may want to play Bowling for Collars, a game designed not only to reduce your collar size but to slim you down in general. You may want to play Run for Your Life, a fast-paced regimen of rigorous exercise that is played nightly at 3 A.M. in New York's Central Park. For the less adventurous there is just plain Walking, which Harry Truman popularized. There is some exercise that will be useful to just about everyone. Find out what yours is and do it!

Take out the garbage!

Children the world over are encouraged by their parents to finish all of the food that is put in front of them. In the United States, children are typically told to finish their food because "children are starving in Europe." By the same obscure logic, children in Europe are told to finish everything on their plates because "children are starving in Asia." And it seems a safe guess that children in Asia are told that "children are starving in Africa" (and the buck doesn't stop there either). Children-are-starving stories are designed to instill guilt in the child who does not finish all of the food he is served.

Some adults have been more affected by such guilt-producing stories than others. People who play the binge game Clean Plate Club are probably those who have been profoundly affected by the early linking of guilt with refusal to eat. The physical capacity of the stomach and not really the appetite is the primary factor in stopping the Club player from eating. Typically, such people will finish not only their own leftovers, but the leftovers of those eating with them. Serving these people smaller portions of food is an effective first step in stopping this binge game from being replayed at every meal. However, it is only a stopgap technique as the player is bound to be exposed to leftovers at restaurants, parties, and other settings where portion sizes cannot be controlled.

Club players and other people who have associated guilt with refusal to eat (or more properly to overeat) must learn a simple, anti-binge Action strategy: Take Out the Garbage! In the beginning you should purposely leave over some food and throw it out just to see that nothing catastrophic happens when you do. Work up to the point where you can throw out unwanted food at will. Learn to substitute the phrase "It is a shame to waste good food" with "It is a shame to waste my life and jeopardize my health by being a human garbage can."

Anti-automation

This Action strategy is for those who work in settings where the horror of tempting vending machines is just steps away. One of my patients frequented a candy machine in her place of business quite often even though she knew it was not healthy for her to do so. In order to break the binging habit she was taught to play Anti-Automation. In this game the patient was required to carry no spare change on her person when she left for work in the morning. She was not to carry more money than she needed for the day if possible (she was allowed to have her credit cards for emergencies). She was also to carry sugar-free hard candies for use in weaning the candy-machine habit. When she felt a strong urge to walk to the machine, she was to walk to the water fountain instead. Most of all, she was encouraged to think of herself, her husband, and her children and how she was jeopardizing her family's welfare by indulging herself in candy (which for this woman was life-threatening).

People who play this game seriously will find that they go through three stages. At Stage 1 they are in the "I want you" stage everytime they pass the candy machine. This stage is characterized by long, soulful gazes at the machine with the eyes focused on the desired treat. Stage 1 lasts about two weeks or so. In Stage 2, they are at the point where they simply look here and there at the machine, but the message, if it were verbalized, is now, "I want you but I can't have you." Stage 2 also lasts about two weeks. Stage 3 is where they walk by the machine and have to remember not to trip over it because it's that unimportant to them. Once they have reached their Moment of Truth and developed a binge-free lifestyle they can live with, Stage 3 should last a lifetime. Then it will be okay to have some candy once in a while. There's nothing wrong with having candy once you are controlling it and it is not controlling you.

Grab bag

One anti-binge Action strategy that seems to work for a good number of my patients is having a "grab bag" on hand. The ingredients of a grab bag are a matter of personal preference but you may want to begin by peeling some carrots, cucumbers, and most any other raw vegetable. Grab Bag is a game that is played when you are still at the stage in the program where you need something you can grab for at times. The game has the element of surprise in that, if you put in a wide enough variety to start, you never know what vegetables you're going to grab out. The greatest surprise, however, comes after you've reached that Moment of Truth in your life and you find that you can painlessly throw away your grab bag and never need it or miss it.

Tag

This is a game you will really enjoy if you have young children in the house. The idea is to tag their food with a name label that is large enough for you to read from a distance. You don't have to tag all of their food, just the sweets or other items you find tempting and know you really shouldn't have. You may want to tag the ice cream, the cookies, the chocolate syrup—anything that might present a problem for you. At some point later on in the program you will no longer feel the need to play Tag since you will have stopped running in circles.

Say "cheese" I

You probably have an old photo of yourself which you really can't stand but you never threw away. It's probably a photo of you at your heaviest, and you may cringe everytime you look at it. Still, one of the reasons you may have held on to that picture is to remind yourself how heavy you once were. But that reminder is doing nothing for you tucked away in the bottom of a chest of drawers. Why not let that photo serve as an incentive to you to take positive action against binging. Put that photo up in some conspicuous place where you (and only you) must look at it everyday. Let it serve as a reminder and an incentive to take action.

Some doctors encourage their overweight patients to play a related game called Looking Glass. In that game, players must look at their nude bodies in a full-length mirror daily. The rationale of Looking Glass is that the patient will become so disgusted with what he sees that he will be highly motivated to change. However, in my clinical experience with many weight patients who have tried Looking Glass, I have found that it seldom works the way the prescribing doctor thought it would. The great danger in this game is that the patient will become very depressed about the way they look and feel helpless to change. Patients look in the mirror and say to themselves, "This is the way I am." However, in Say "Cheese," patients are afforded the opportunity of saying, "This is the way I *was*"—even if the photo was taken only a week ago!

Say "cheese" II

After a month or so of playing Say "Cheese" I, advance to Say "Cheese" II. In this sequel, the object is to hang a photo of yourself at your thinnest next to your Say "Cheese" I photo. You may find that you spend more time gazing at your thin photo than the other; that's okay provided you look at *both* each day. To prevent the pictures from becoming merely part of the woodwork, rotate their placement in your house or apartment on a weekly basis. Now you have both positive and negative motivators working to get you where you want to be!

Taking a dip

You've just been invited to a party where you know there will be a tempting array of hors d'oeuvres. If it's appropriate to do so (that is, if the party's in someone's house and not a catered affair), you could call the host or hostess and ask if it would be okay to bring some raw vegetables and a homemade diet dip. Green peppers, mushrooms, carrots, celery, etc., are sure to be greatly appreciated by your host or hostess if such diet hors d'oeuvres have not already been planned. If, for some reason, it is not possible for you to Take a Dip, and there won't be any food at the party that you can eat, why not leave over some extra calories from your last meal to use at the party (or simply eat before going and do some extra-heavy mingling and relating while there).

Hospitality personality

Some people will not leave other people alone at parties and social gatherings. Pushy hosts and hostesses, even other guests, will keep hounding you to take a taste of this or a sip of that. Sometimes it seems they will just not take "No" for an answer. There are many different ways to respond to the pushy host or hostess. One is to passively accept and swallow whatever is being dished out. Experienced players of Gin Dummy are well versed in that mode of responding. Another alternative is to become verbally abusive or even violently aggressive to the person doing the offering. That alternative is frowned upon for important business lunches (and for all other occasions as well) for a variety of reasons.

The Action response to the pushy host or hostess is to play Hospitality Personality. The ultimate goal of the player is to be able to assertively refuse to be bulldozed into having a food or drink that he really does not want. In practice, some of my patients have found it too difficult to simply say "No" when they first begin playing Hospitality Personality. As stopgaps along the way to a genuinely assertive future, they have found excuses like "Thank you, I'll have some later" and "No thank you, I have an upset stomach" useful. The Hospitality Personality game ends once the player can say "No" to a food offering without feeling guilty.

Speak your piece

People want respect. They want to know they are being listened to when they speak, and they want to know that what they have to say is important. Whether you are fat, thin, or in between, it would be helpful to get into the habit of doing your share of the speaking without feeling self-conscious or that what you say has to be perfect. One of my obese patients always had a difficult time speaking at PTA meetings. She had good ideas, but she was afraid to stand up and express them because of her weight. She felt that all of the other people in the room would just look at her weight instead of listening to what she had to say. She thought they might say to themselves, "How smart can she be if she's so fat?" or "What right does fatso have to talk?" It was not until this woman began to speak her piece that an upward spiral of self-esteem began to develop.

LSD trip
(Long, Satisfying, Diet-conscious trip)

The value of a vacation and a change cannot be overstated. If you can get away and not make food the highlight of your trip, you will probably come back feeling a lot better about yourself. Take a long trip (three weeks if feasible) and do everything to make it as satisfying as possible. Try to avoid staying with relatives or even friends if doing so will make you sacrifice some of your independence with respect to eating habits. Be diet-conscious throughout your trip but don't be obsessed with your diet. Remember: You can have virtually anything you want *in moderation*. Vacations are also great times to begin lifelong exercise habits—something you should give some serious thought to while you are away. Experimentation with different eating/exercise habits is the key to a successful LSD Trip.

Home-base ball

If you think of frankfurters when you think of baseball, this anti-binge Action game is for you. The game begins when you discover new and exciting things to do around the house. Use your imagination but please, no whipped cream—farmer's cheese is okay if you must. The idea of this game is to "have a ball" at your homebase without making food the highlight of the game.

Chicken!

Originally a game played by two motor vehicles speeding toward each other or toward some precipice, this game is played slightly differently today: baked instead of fried. Play often and don't forget the soup if you get the sniffles.

Go fish!

Like chicken, this is a good game to play baked.

Hot potato!

There's nothing wrong with this game baked either. Just go easy on the butter, margarine, and/or sour cream.

Spin the bottle

The idea of this game is not to become half-baked.

Orange bowl

Have one filled with oranges and other fruits at all times.

Happy D-A-E-S

A patient of mine had some success with the Action component of her program by switching around the order of the dishes she served at dinner. She was happiest with dessert (D) first, appetizer (A) next, followed by the entree (E), and then something hot, like soup (S) or coffee. Interestingly, some scientific evidence could probably be mustered to support why this style of eating was helpful. Sugar enters the bloodstream faster than either fats or proteins, and it is therefore conceivable that this woman experienced a sense of fullness earlier by eating dessert first (of course, she may have been better off not eating dessert at all, but that's another matter). Also, hot liquids at the end of a meal seem to promote a sense of fullness.

Although I cannot wholeheartedly endorse Happy D-A-E-S as an Action game that everyone should try, I mention it because it seemed to have been of help to one of my patients. What is one person's meat is another's placebo . . . or something like that.

Follow the leader

The AAA method of binge-breaking described in this book is designed to help you learn to be slim, accept yourself slim, and become a slim person. To do so, you may need some "on-the-job training" before you get there. In training to become a slim person, it is a good idea to play Follow the Leader: spend a day, a week, a month—as long as you can—with a slim person. If you don't have a slim person you can stay with, rent one from a model agency or local rent-a-secretary agency. Spend all the time you can with her. Go shopping with her, and at lunch order exactly what she orders (even if you can't stand zucchini). Throughout your training period take note of the attention the opposite sex gives your "leader," and discuss how she responds to such attention. Really listen to what slim people talk about and observe how their lives do not seem to revolve around food. When playing Follow the Leader remember: There is nothing so contagious as example.

Tight places, smiling faces

When you are overweight there are some places, such as seats on public buses, that may fit you very snugly if at all. Right now when you sit down in one of those places or try to walk through one of those doorways, all kinds of negative feelings may be aroused. The object of Tight Places, Smiling Faces is to change all of that. The game is played by genuinely smiling when you settle down in or pass through any of those tight places. You smile, secure in the knowledge that you will one day be able to fit easily. This game should be played again when you are down to your goal weight. That is, purposely ride a public conveyance or walk through a doorway that was previously too tight and smile, knowing that you attained the goal you set out to reach.

Bathing beauty but no contest

Part of anti-binge Action is accepting your body as part of you. This means that you shouldn't deprive yourself of anything solely on the basis of the way your body looks. As a case in point consider how you look in a bathing suit. Many of my obese patients won't even put on a bathing suit because they feel they look so silly in one. Yet many of these patients would like to go to the beach or to a pool and swim. I advise them to do so and in so doing accept themselves for who they are now and look forward to the day when they will feel even more comfortable in a swimsuit. *The local pool or beach doesn't have to be a place for a bathing-beauty contest unless you choose to make it one.* For some patients, going bathing in public is a harrowing experience; they think everyone is commenting on how ridiculous they look. Even if everyone were making those comments (and they're probably not)—so what? Is that a reflection on them or you? The idea of Bathing Beauty But No Contest is not to let your poor body image get in the way of your life. The contest ends once you've begun to accept your arms, legs, thighs, stomach—all of you.

Person to person

Clinical experience has shown me that overweight people can profit tremendously from relating to others on a deep, one-to-one level. It is, in some respects, the lack of such heart-to-heart relating that promotes hand-to-mouth relating. To play Person to Person, find someone to relate to and set aside about forty minutes per meeting to "relate." Let "relate" mean anything you want it to, just make sure to look into each other's eyes and not talk about trivial or everyday kinds of things. You will be surprised to find what effect this simple action exercise can have on your attitude toward yourself and food.

Simon says

Have you ever had your hair cut in a highly flattering way, gotten dressed up, looked great, and then had your spouse not even notice? One patient of mine who looked and felt smashing just before she and her husband were off to a wedding took Action when her husband was preoccupied with finding the car keys instead of being preoccupied with her. This woman found that a slightly modified version of Simon Says did wonders in conditioning her husband to take notice when notice was due and to compliment her when a compliment was in order (he had always been willing to put her down at the drop of a hat). After her husband failed to notice her new hair-do, her new dress, and how generally lovely she looked, she physically backed him up against the wall and looked him straight in the eye. The following dialogue ensued:

WIFE: We are going to play Simon Says. Now, Simon Says to say, "My honey, you look great!"

HUSBAND: My honey, you look great!

WIFE: Simon Says say, "Your hair looks great, that dress looks terrific on you. You're the beautiful woman I married.

HUSBAND: Your hair looks great, that dress looks terrific on you. You're the beautiful woman I married.

WIFE: Thank you. You say the nicest things!

Some might argue that my patient should have been content with herself and not care about what her husband did or did not say. Although there is some validity to this point of view, the fact is this woman *did* care whether or not her husband noticed her. Playing Simon Says served her needs and got her the acknowledgment she desired.

Because I'm worth it

In this Action game an increased amount of time is spent rewarding and pleasuring yourself because you're worth it. After-all, if you aren't going to reward and pleasure yourself, who will? Go to the beauty parlor, buy a new outfit—enjoy life! If anyone asks why you are suddenly doing these things, the answer should be clear enough: *Because you're worth it!* Once you begin to act it, you will begin to really feel and believe that you *are* worth it, once you begin to really feel and believe that you are worth it, self-destructive acts will fall by the wayside and a bright, binge-free future will be in the offing.

Blind man's brush

Some people report that when a binge "comes over" them, all they can see is food and they go blind to anything and everything in the environment. One stopgap, anti-binge strategy is to brush your teeth when this desire to binge comes over you. Brushing your teeth is not only good for your teeth and a very healthy competing activity for eating, but it will also serve to alter the taste of some foods that you may want to binge on just after brushing. Experiment with different toothpastes to see which alters your taste for food the most. You may also want to try some of the powders on the market for cleaning teeth; they really taste awful and will serve your purpose well.

Out of bounds

In this game, a section of your pantry is walled off and declared out of bounds to you. Foods that other members of your family might want are to be stored there, but for you that area is absolutely forbidden. You might remember that in the Awareness game of Fencing you did something similar. However, that was just for the purpose of helping you to gain an awareness. Now it is absolutely forbidden to violate the boundary line you set up. Make an agreement with your spouse, or whoever, that pantry raiding by you in the out of bounds area is not to be tolerated and is to be enforced with strict penalties.

Donate your old body to science

You don't really have to donate your old *body* to science, just your old clothes to some charitable organization. Make a point of visiting that organization at least once a month to donate something. Go public with your weight loss—tell people you are dieting and that you expect to lose even more weight in the future (and will donate more clothes). Hiding the fact that you are dieting may make it too easy for you to revert to binging ways that are better kept in your past.

Psychological judo

This is a mental Action game designed to help you to "go with the force" rather than against it. Suppose, for example, you have been able to keep to your anti-binge program for months and this invitation finds its way to your mailbox:

YOU'RE INVITED TO A PARTY!
DON'T BRING ANYTHING BUT YOUR APPETITE!
FESTIVITIES BEGIN AT 5 . . . FEASTING BEGINS AT 6.

An invitation like this is certainly inviting! If you've been on the program and doing well you may be bothered by such temptation. Further, you may start wondering about what types of food will be served. And after you wonder a while about that, you might say to yourself, "I'll never be thin. All I think about is food!"

Here it would seem that some Psychological Judo is in order. The idea here is to "go with" the thought of food and not try to fight it. Why get down on yourself for thinking about food when an invitation is so clearly designed to guide your thinking in that direction. Instead, think about the food and how great it will be to taste a little of this and a little of that without going overboard as you did in the past. Psychological Judo is a game you must learn to play if you are to restructure your life. When it comes to designing a binge-free future for yourself, Psychological Judo is an infinitely more powerful game than Boxing-Off Urges.

On your side

In this Action strategy you resolve once and for all that you are not going to be on Tony's side, on Ellen's side, on anyone's side but your own. This does not in any way mean that you are going to become selfish, unfeeling, unsympathetic, or insensitive to the needs of others. What it does mean is that you are going to put yourself in touch with your own needs and effectively act on them. If you want to eat certain healthy foods for dinner, you will have to take *your* side and refuse to eat in a fast food restaurant—despite the fact your husband has a yen to do so. If you want to go out socially more often or travel or engage in any number of activities, you will have to take *your* side and take steps toward doing what you want to do.

Being on your side means being assertive, a skill that is quite useful in many aspects of binge-breaking. What is being suggested here is that you can be responsive to the needs of others without ignoring your own needs. Assertion need not be aggression, just as self-interest need not be selfishness. Remember: If you are not on your side, your side is going to be pretty empty!

Breaking the binge:

Attitude change

The final stage of the AAA binge-breaking program is Attitude change. Your Awareness training has taught you that a binge is not like a knee jerk; it is not a reflex. A binge is a state of mind that may be brought on by the people around you, the place you are in, the time of day, or any number of other factors. Your use of the Action strategies described in Chapter 5 have shown that you can rob food of its control over you and make problem eating one less problem in your life. Your task now is to *maintain* the benefits you've derived from the Awareness and Action skills you have learned. In short, what is required now is a change in past attitudes and behaviors toward yourself and toward food, and the development of a binge-free lifestyle you can live with for the rest of your life. Toward that goal we now offer some thoughts on the perils of change, the "foodaholic" myth, and the concept we have been referring to as the "Moment of Truth."

The perils of change

Change can be exciting. It can also be frightening . . . *very* frightening. One consequence of anti-binge Awareness and Action is change in ourselves, not only in our physical appearance but in the way we feel about ourselves and the way we must respond to others. We see ourselves in a new light and that newness frequently reveals something we may not have been aware of or something we prefer not to think about. Others see us in a new light, too, and we must be prepared to deal with their attraction, defensiveness, jealousy, and other responses that the change is sure to evoke. Change means discriminating negative bodily states and dealing with them appropriately—not just turning to food as the panacea. Change may signal competition (in employment, in wardrobe, in social relations, etc.) where we have shunned it in the past. Change may result in the development of a healthy self-esteem. But with that self-esteem comes the duties and obligations of a person who feels worthy, effective, respectable, loved, and needed: *You can no longer rely on food in troubled times, you must rely on yourself.*

The "foodaholic" myth

One way of dealing with the perils of change is to deny that any change has taken place. This is what the notion of "foodaholism" seeks to do: deny that you will ever be able to transform yourself from one who is controlled by food to one who is in control. Like the alcoholic who views himself as a person who must never take a drink again, so the foodaholic declares prohibition on certain foods and swears off them forever.

There is no doubt that many people with drinking problems have profited greatly by declaring themselves to be alcoholics and abstaining from liquor for the rest of their lives. However, it is impossible to abstain from food for one week (and inadvisable to abstain for even one day), let alone the rest of your life. Even to say that you are going to abstain from eating only certain foods (e.g., all ice cream, cake, and candy) is probably unrealistic as you have been eating these foods since early childhood and you will be exposed to them daily. The result of making an idle promise to abstain from such foods for the rest of your life leads to an inevitable breach of that promise and a consequential loss of self-respect. After you've sworn off all chocolate and then tasted two chocolate-covered raisins you might say to yourself, "I don't even have the self-control and

the willpower to keep away from two chocolate-covered raisins.
. . . How will I ever have the self-control and the willpower to
accomplish anything important?"

Foodaholism is a catchy idea, but it is an idea that runs
counter to everything the AAA binge-breaking program stands
for. At best, foodaholism is a notion that can be of very limited
use in keeping you away from certain foods for a limited time
period. At worst, foodaholism is a destructive notion that can
put you at war with food and cause you to fight a "battle of the
binge" every moment you are in the vicinity of appealing foods.
Of course, if there was a single shred of scientifically acceptable evidence to prove that the approach worked—if it could be
demonstrated that foodaholics who swear off certain foods are
able to live happily in total abstinence, and achieve and maintain goal weights—I would be convinced of its efficacy and use
such an approach with all of my patients. As it stands now,
foodaholism is a highly destructive notion, destructive for at
least five reasons:

1. *"Foodaholism" equates overeating with disease, and overeating is not a disease.* The person who frequently overeats
   may appear *as if* he is suffering from some disease though,
   in reality, he isn't. Where is the gene or chromosome which
   dictates that you must consume a half gallon of frozen yogurt per week? Have you ever caught foodaholism after a
   foodaholic sneezed? The point is, as far as modern science
   can determine, there is no disease called foodaholism.*

2. *"Foodaholism" denies the opportunity for growth to people
   with problem eating habits.* "You may be 'well' now but there
   is always the potential of becoming ill." When you believe

---

* Similar arguments have been made against the notion of alcoholism as
a disease. See, for example, Craig MacAndrew's article, "On the Notion
that Certain Persons Who Are Given to Frequent Drunkenness Suffer from
a Disease Called Alcoholism" in S.C. Plog and R.B. Edgerton (*Eds.*),
Changing Perspectives in Mental Illness, New York: Holt, Rinehart and
Winston, 1969.

in foodaholism, you believe that you may become "ill" at any time. But doesn't it make more sense to view problem eating as a bad habit that can be gotten rid of? Must all thumb-suckers be "thumbsuckeraholics"? Must all nailbiters be "nailbiteraholics"? Don't we, as human beings, have the potential for growth?

3. *"Foodaholism" provides a convenient crutch for returning to binging ways.* The person who views himself a foodaholic has a pat, ever-ready excuse for binging just about any time of the day. He can simply say, "Just as a drug addict needs his 'fix' and an alcoholic needs his drink, so I need my pistachio ice cream."

4. *"Foodaholism" shrouds Awareness strategies in a negative light.* Foodaholics are condemned to living their lives dwelling on what once was problem eating habit. Awareness strategies like *Person*al Touch are foreign to the foodaholic who must daily focus and dwell on his awareness of himself as a person with a problem.

5. *"Foodaholism" shrouds Action strategies in a negative light.* For the foodaholic, every waking moment is a battle against becoming ill. Counter to AAA binge-breaking principles as expressed in *Person*al Touch and *Person*al Growth, all actions taken with respect to food by foodaholics are designed to restrain, resist, prohibit, inhibit, quell, restrict, hold back, and hold in. Moreover, while the binge-breaker's actions designed to modify food intake are clearly designed to be *stopgap* strategies, foodaholic "strategies" are long-term and they condemn their users to being mobilized for battle their entire lives. To put it another way, the binge-breaker is moving *toward* a lifestyle he can live with, while the foodaholic spends his life running *away* from a lifestyle he can't live with.

If you are truly sincere about making problem eating a problem of your past, it is time to stop believing in the myth of foodaholism. If you are ready to acknowledge that you have the capacity for growth, you are ready to stop clinging to foodaholic balderdash like, "I am never more than one bite away from a binge." If you are ready to renounce pessimism for the challenge of optimism, to let action and awareness work for you instead of against you, you are ready to break free of the chains of the foodaholic philosophy. You are not addicted to food; you need it to live. You should be able to love food—not avoid it like the plague. You don't have to spend every day of your life feeling deprived and/or guilty; you have a right to feel as "normal" as the next person. *You can have any food you want*—in moderation.

Living binge-free

Beyond weight loss and the control of compulsive eating habits, the AAA binge-breaking program is designed to help put you in control of your *life*. Frankly, I believe the AAA program is not for everyone. In fact, it is probably not for most people, for most people want and seem to need to be controlled.* When it comes to dieting, people want to be told what to eat and drink for breakfast, lunch, and dinner. They seek out "miracle" drugs, powders, potions, and diets in their frenzied search for a foolproof method of avoiding conscious choice and meaningful change in their attitudes and behaviors.

The good news is that because binging is a state of mind, the power to become binge-free is within everyone's grasp! Bingers have a choice. On the one hand, they can spend the rest of their waking lives enjoying sporadic binging and suffering through sporadic dieting. On the other, they can seriously go about using the Awareness and Action strategies described in

* See, for example, Erich Fromm's classic work on this subject, *Escape from Freedom*, New York: Holt, Rinehart and Winston, 1941.

this book and resolve to make a change—a most exciting but potentially frightening change—in their lives. The change will involve not only dealing with food effectively, but dealing with *life* effectively. Instead of turning to food in times of anxiety, stress, boredom, anger, and fatigue they will identify these feelings and deal with them effectively—*just as an effective, worthy, respectable, loved, and needed* person would deal with them.

The moment of truth

You may be one of those people who feel helpless in fending off a binge despite a keen awareness of your eating habits and a working knowledge of anti-binge Action strategies. If so, your overeating and binging habits are probably serving some purpose in your life. That is, in addition to being a conditioned reaction to stress of some sort, your binging may be serving some "grander" purpose in the "grand scheme of things." You may, for example, be keeping extra weight on to shield you from attention from the opposite sex. I have referred to the instant a person gets in touch with the unconscious reason he or she has been binging as a "Moment of Truth"; a kind of day of reckoning with food. It is the day you find out what it is you want and why you have been playing Slack Off, Trampoline, Giant Steps, and related binge games. Moreover—if it is a day when you resolve to put your Awareness and Action strategies to work for you—it is the point at which food no longer dictates to you, rules you, calls you, or hovers over you.

In practice, what we are calling a "Moment of Truth" need not be a "moment" in the traditional sense. It may be more of a *process* whereby you

· become aware of the reasons you have been unable to lose weight in the past;

· take action to develop a more adaptive lifestyle; and

· effectively change your attitudes and behaviors for the better.

What is a Moment of Truth like? The following case histories describe what it was like for some of my patients.

CASE 1   This patient's Moment of Truth came as a result of the use of the What's-Wrong-With-This-Picture? technique. In a state of deep hypnosis the patient was able to visualize herself thin, but there was something very wrong with the picture. . . . She had no friends! In this patient's mind, being slim had somehow become associated with being sophisticated, snobbish, and "uppity." The patient liked to view herself and her close friends as "earthy" people who were not particularly sophisticated and who didn't care to be. This patient's Moment of Truth culminated in a commitment to break her mental association between "slim" and "sophisticated." She went forward in her program assured that if her loss of weight would mean the loss of friends, they were not friends worth having in the first place.

CASE 2   A Moment of Truth in this patient's life came when she realized that every time she lost weight her husband became extraordinarily flirtatious with other women and probably engaged in extramarital affairs. The patient was a very attractive woman who was married to a successful but emotionally immature, juvenile, and extremely insecure man. As long as the patient remained obese, there was peace in the marriage. However, whenever the woman lost weight and started looking good, the husband became extremely jealous and began to believe that all male attention was being focused on his wife. The consequence was that this man would then attempt to "retaliate" by attempting to prove to his wife (and to himself) that he too was attractive to the opposite sex. He did so by seeking attention from any eligible female and by a lot of extramarital dating—revealed through many telltale signs.

This patient had a dilemma. She believed that if she lost weight the only thing she could do to keep her husband from straying would be to constantly "feed his ego" and reassure him of her devotion. The husband staunchly refused to be seen in therapy saying he knew more than the therapist. In her Moment of Truth, the patient resolved to lose the weight and then deal with her husband's problems. She was not going to let his problems interfere with her living a full, slim, and binge-free life.

CASE 3   This patient was a fifty-seven-year-old widow who had gained an inordinate amount of weight after the death of her husband. Early in therapy, when the patient was considering how she would feel if she did go ahead and have sexual relations with someone new, the patient said, "What if a man I meet looks at the body of a fifty-seven-year-old fat person and says 'Yeccchh!'" Later on in therapy this patient realized that she was remaining a fifty-seven-year-old *fat* person *because* of her ambivalence toward approaching sexual relations with someone other than her husband. Although she did crave the emotional closeness that comes with sexual intercourse, lifelong notions about the inappropriateness of premarital and nonmarital intercourse prevented this woman from achieving that closeness. It was not until this woman worked through her parentally induced sexual hangups that she was able to come to her Moment of Truth and begin to salvage her emotions, her figure—her life.

CASE 4   This patient was a middle-aged woman who had an obese adolescent daughter. The patient felt very guilty about her daughter's obesity both because she thought she had given the girl "bad genes" and because she had deprived her of sweets while growing up (and in that way making sweets all the more attractive outside of the house).

In her Moment of Truth the patient realized that she had been unable to lose weight in the past because she felt to do so would somehow be "deserting" her daughter. At one point the patient said, "How can I leave her alone?" Finally, the patient began to realize that keeping her own weight high was not a rational method of helping, consoling, or showing empathy for her daughter. She came to strongly believe that the best way she could help her daughter was by modeling effective means of weight loss—and that meant awareness, action, and an entire change in attitude and behavior.

CASE 5   Like many patients before a Moment of Truth has been reached, this patient had gone up and down in weight for years. A binge almost always occurred just as she was beginning to look good and to get male attention. The binge would last for days; when it was over, the effects of months of dieting had been totally wiped out.

The patient's problem revolved around a classic psychological reason for obesity: She was deathly afraid of sexual intercourse and pregnancy and ate to ward off male attention. Her fear was so great that she even felt uncomfortable and anxious around women in their late months of pregnancy. By remaining obese for the majority of her life, this patient had successfully warded off any male sexual attraction. Her Moment of Truth came when she resolved to work through her problems with male attraction while once and for all bringing her weight down to a manageable level.

CASE 6   Using the What's-Wrong-With-This-Picture? technique, this patient blushed when she visualized herself thin. In her scene she was clad in attractive, sexy, scanty underclothing, and there were numerous men looking at her admiringly. After the visualization the patient remarked that she had always been faithful to her husband and had always wanted to be faithful to her husband. However, in her Moment of Truth, this patient realized that somewhere deep inside her there was a longing for experience with a variety of men—experience she had never had. Unlike many weight patients who harbor inner fears of sexual intimacy, this patient harbored a fear of promiscuity. Losing weight made her *feel* sexier; this bothered her and feelings of guilt, worthlessness, and shame welled up inside her. Psychotherapy was designed to work through these feelings.

CASE 7 Ever since this patient read *Wuthering Heights,* she associated weight loss with death. In therapy, this patient recalled how affected she had been by the death of Catherine— "she 'faded away' from consumption (tuberculosis) and died." Every time this patient succeeded in taking off a lot of weight, she would be deeply affected by her friends' innocent kidding remarks like "you're fading away" or "you're becoming emaciated." This patient could only think of lifelong slimness as a way of life when she was helped toward equating loss of weight with life, not death.

CASE 8 Through her high school and college years, this patient believed that if she lost weight she would become more active athletically, socially, and sexually. She felt that if she became more active in these areas, her grades would decline and her life would be in shambles. In graduate school, this irrational belief not only persisted but was compounded. Specifically, the patient was the only female in a study group. She believed that her weight made possible a friendly, working relationship with the men in the study group.

As a working professional, this patient continued to believe her excess weight facilitated businesslike relationships with the opposite sex and helped her avoid activities that would impair her professional effectiveness. Additionally, she believed any weight loss would be threatening to her male, nonsexual friends and jeopardize her friendship with them. Until this patient came to a Moment of Truth in her life, she would not have been a good candidate for any weight-reduction program.

CASE 9 "How will I deal with adverse happenings in my life if I don't binge?" and "Will I become a drug addict? an alcoholic?" are only some of the questions this patient would ask herself nightly. A deathly fear of giving up food as a "pacifier" haunted this patient. She needed to be convinced that a binge-free lifestyle was a possibility and the solution would not be worse than the problem.

CASE 10   This patient was born with a rare intestinal disease. In infancy and in early childhood she was extremely underweight and gaunt. For that entire period of her life, the patient recalls, "It would do my mother's heart good for me to binge . . . her greatest joy in life was watching me eat and eat and eat." Subsequently, in adolescence, this patient had not only achieved her proper weight but had become obese. Still, her parents—over-reactive to any signs of weight loss—always seemed to be encouraging her to eat more than she really had to. Additionally, they would tell her things like, "It doesn't matter what you look like on the outside, it's whats inside that counts" when she would complain about being too heavy. At some point in her life she developed the notion that only "special people" (like her family) would be able to "see beyond" her fat. In therapy, our task was to help her to realize she no longer had to overeat to please others; she had to eat normally to please herself.

CASE 11   This patient grew up in a highly restrictive home environment where all her food intake was closely monitored. Her parents owned a dress manufacturing company in New York City's garment district and more than anything else, they wanted to shower their daughter with fashionable creations. The patient, however, in an apparent rebellion against her parents' wishes, rejected the chic clothing and ate all the more. She would binge while out of the house and occasionally even sneak food into the house. The patient was quite successful in defying her parents. Her task in therapy was to un-do the damage she had done to herself.

CASE 12   This patient's Moment of Truth involved her sense of humor* which she felt was too cynical, sarcastic, and "catty" as regards her coworkers and friends. In the patient's own words, she possessed a "thin person's wit." She believed that her rather hostile sense of humor had potential for disrupting some of her friendships and that her excess weight was there to

---

* Or, perhaps more accurately, her "sense of rage."

keep her sense of humor from coming out. As long as this patient remained obese, she could not feel comfortable about ridiculing anyone or expressing the contemptuous thoughts she was feeling; all of the rage and hostility were sealed behind a wall of fat. As a result, this patient feared that if she lost weight, her interpersonal relationships would suffer.

CASE 13   During the course of psychotherapy, this patient came to realize that something dreadful had happened to her every time she lost weight. The first time she lost and kept off weight she started dating a dentist with whom she wound up in a car accident. The second time she was able to lose weight and keep it off for a while she was fired by her boss with whom she had begun to have an affair. Just before beginning treatment, the patient had ended a passionate but stormy relationship with a man; a relationship which included one suicide attempt on the part of her lover and, at the very end of the affair, an abortion. Subsequently, the patient resolutely "swore off" men (and weight loss) saying, "I can't let myself get hurt like that again." Clearly, therapy for this patient involved much more than the mere loss of weight.

CASE 14   This patient promised herself she would lose weight only after she had undergone plastic surgery to alter the shape of her nose. After two operations the patient was still dissatisfied with her physical appearance despite the fact that friends unanimously agreed that the surgery had been successful. This patient's resistance to anti-binge Awareness and Action strategies could be summed up by her own words, "No matter how much weight I lose, it doesn't matter; I will always be ugly!"

CASE 15   In his younger days, this patient had been a "jock" who was physically active, handsomely built, and a BMOC* in the right way. In his Moment of Truth, the patient

* Big Man on Campus (in this sense referring to popularity not size).

realized that his excess weight was an expression of hostility against his wife, a woman who had married him (he thought) because he was captain of the school football team. Soon after the marriage the patient began to gain a lot of weight in a relatively short period of time. His wife protested and begged him to slim down. However, for this patient, gaining weight amounted to his giving his wife the message that if she really loved him she would love him fat as well as slim, he wasn't going to live up to anyone's expectations but his own.

CASE 16   This patient's Moment of Truth revolved around her extreme fear that her life would not change at all after she took off the excess pounds her binging had put on. The patient felt she would have no place to go, nothing to get dressed up for, and really no one to go anywhere with. In her Moment of Truth she resolved to lose weight and work toward independence and constructive assertiveness that would see her through to her goal weight. Further, she would use these newfound skills to bring activities and joy into her life.

CASE 17   In her Moment of Truth this patient discovered that she had been unable to lose weight in the past because she felt that any weight loss amounted to a "deception." Feeling basically inadequate, this patient had used her weight to advertise and alert others to her supposed inadequacy as a human being. Losing weight would then amount to "pulling the wool" over everyone's eyes and disguising her basic lack of worth. In other areas of her life this patient also believed that she had been successfully fooling people and that sooner or later it was all going to be uncovered. This patient was able to make good progress in her program when these irrational beliefs were properly dispelled.

CASE 18   This patient's Moment of Truth came when she was able to accept the fact that, in her case, a search for "deep-rooted" or "unconscious" reasons for her inability to lose weight would be a futile search. This patient had been in psychoanalysis for a number of years with a competent psychoanalyst. When I first saw her I noted that she had already acquired a great deal of insight into her presenting problem. What she lacked were action strategies and an "I can do it this time" attitude. Despite the fact that this patient had tremendous insight into her problem eating habits, the patient persisted in believing that her analyst had overlooked some important deep-rooted reason for her overeating and binging behavior. On many occasions she told me, "there's something that has not been brought to the surface."

After seeing this patient for quite some time and after obtaining a careful history of her treatment with the analyst, my conclusion was that this patient's search for the missing deep-rooted factor was a cop-out. I tried to impress upon her the fact that whether there was or was not a missing link was irrelevant at this point. What we had to do was follow not the "right" or "wrong" method of correcting her eating habits, but the *most useful* method. In other words, she may have been right that some intrapsychic factor had been overlooked. Then again she may have been wrong. But regardless, more insight would not have helped this woman. Eating Awareness, Action strategies, and a positive Attitude *could* help her. And all she needed to begin to become binge-free was to give up saying, "I wish I could find that mysterious reason why I eat" and begin saying, "I am going to become aware of my eating habtis, I am going to take positive action to correct them, and I'm going to do it this time because I want to lose weight."

If you have had a problem with food and with yourself in the past, ask yourself now:

· What's my Moment of Truth?
· Am I ready to stop playing games with myself and those around me?
· Can I see the light at the end of the tunnel?

· If I can't see the light, what obstacles are in the way?
· How can I use the Awareness and Action strategies described in this book to break down those obstacles?
· What other strategies can I use to break down those obstacles?

Not everyone will be able to come up with satisfactory answers to the difficult questions posed above. If you think you could use help in finding the answers you shouldn't be ashamed to seek the assistance of a psychologist or other mental health professional to help you toward your Moment of Truth, to guide you and enhance your Awareness training, to teach you effective Action strategies, to help you mold for yourself a binge-free lifestyle you can live with.

A final note

Hopefully, your Awareness training and the Action strategies herein have provided you with the tools for a binge-breaking attitude/behavior change and a binge-free life. Hopefully, you have been prompted to begin thinking about what your Moment of Truth might be. Hopefully, you can see—more clearly than ever before—the absurdity of fad dieting; the silliness of eating from a highly regimented list of foods; the imbecility of drinking inordinate amounts of water or other, more exotic potions; the unrealistic, almost magical quality of thinking that goes, "If I can only stay on this diet, I will change my life." Hopefully, you have acquired the insight to see that the quick, *temporary* weight loss you achieve with fad diets amounts only to a brief pat on the back, a pat that will inevitably be followed by a slap in the face. Hopefully, you are ready to accept the fact that no "miracle" diet program, potion, or pill can provide you with the self-awareness you so desperately need to make a meaningful change in your life. Hopefully, the message of this book has been received and indelibly etched in your brain: *The only way to permanent control of problem eating and permanent weight loss is a lifestyle change, not a diet. You are* not *a foodaholic!* It is within your power to live a binge-free, "normal" existence or a binge-laden struggle: *the choice is yours.*

A binge is a state of mind, not a state of hunger. You know there have been times when you felt so "right" about yourself you actually had to remind yourself to eat. Once you have completed and benefited from your Awareness training, learned and practiced your Action strategies, and succeeded in positively changing your attitudes and behaviors, that feeling of basic "rightness" will become a daily occurrence rather than an exceptional event. The dividends pay off in terms of a slimmer, healthier, sexier, more sociable and self-confident you whom you can accept, live with, and even love. A you who is no longer afraid to make a change for the better in your life. A you who can go anywhere you want, eat anything you like, and still not lose sight of the new lifestyle you are going to maintain. A you who deep in your heart has learned that all the food in the world cannot make you feel as good as you can make yourself feel.